Living with Diabetes and Uncertainty in Cairo

Living with Diabetes and Uncertainty in Cairo offers an ethnographic exploration of the interactions of two different understandings of type-2 diabetes: one related to the notion of *ḍaghṭ*, translated as "pressure" or "stress," and another related primarily to obesity. The book is set in Egypt but draws links to a diabetes clinic in Denmark and a multinational medical company, as well as engaging with international diabetes research and guidelines. It tells a story of uncertainty, not only among people in Cairo, but also within medical research, and considers what uncertainty may generate in both bodies and societies at large. The chapters provide valuable insight into the lives of those in Cairo who are diagnosed with type-2 diabetes, and explore how those lives are linked to global movements. The book ultimately reflects on the question of what is overlooked and why in prevention strategies and treatments of type-2 diabetes in Egypt. It will be of particular interest to scholars of anthropology, global and public health, and the Middle East and North Africa.

Mille Kjærgaard Thorsen is an Assistant Professor in the School of Social Work at VIA University College in Aarhus, Denmark, where she teaches and conducts research in the cross-fields of health and social studies. She holds a PhD from the Department of Anthropology at Aarhus University.

Routledge Studies in Health and Medical Anthropology

Affective Health and Masculinities in South Africa
An Ethnography of (In)vulnerability
Hans Reihling

Wandering the Wards
An Ethnography of Hospital Care and its Consequences for People Living with Dementia
Katie Featherstone, Andy Northcott

Actively Dying
The Creation of Muslim Identities through End-of-Life Care in the United States
Cortney Hughes Rinker

amaXhosa Circumcision
Stories of Manhood and Mental Health
Lauraine M. H. Vivian

Treating Heroin Addiction in Norway
The Pharmaceutical Other
Aleksandra Bartoszko

Childlessness in Bangladesh
Intersectionality, Suffering and Resilience
Papreen Nahar

Negotiating the Pandemic
Cultural, National, and Individual Constructions of COVID-19
Edited by Inayat Ali and Robbie Davis-Floyd

Living with Diabetes and Uncertainty in Cairo

Sweetness Under Pressure

Mille Kjærgaard Thorsen

Routledge
Taylor & Francis Group
LONDON AND NEW YORK

First published 2023
by Routledge
4 Park Square, Milton Park, Abingdon, Oxon OX14 4RN

and by Routledge
605 Third Avenue, New York, NY 10158

Routledge is an imprint of the Taylor & Francis Group, an informa business

British Library Cataloguing-in-Publication Data
A catalogue record for this book is available from the British Library

Library of Congress Cataloging-in-Publication Data
A catalog record has been requested for this book

ISBN: 978-1-032-32866-9 (hbk)
ISBN: 978-1-032-35618-1 (pbk)
ISBN: 978-1-003-32768-4 (ebk)

Typeset in Sabon
by Deanta Global Publishing Services, Chennai, India

Contents

Acknowledgments

I dedicate this book, first and foremost, to everyone in Cairo who contributed their time and friendship during my months of fieldwork. A heart-felt thank you to the families who opened their homes and hearts.

Thank you also to all of the doctors, pharmacists, dieticians, nurses, and other healthcare personnel who crossed my path in Cairo, and who agreed to participate in interviews and/or allowed me to conduct participant observation studies in their clinics and hospitals. I realize that my questions and presence were not always easy. I owe much of this book to your expertise and support. A special thank you also to all of the people who passed through these clinics as patients, and who shared their experiences and stories with me. In addition, I wish to thank the Novo Nordisk office and employees in Cairo for agreeing to assist with – but also participate in – my research. For this I am forever grateful.

I further wish to thank patients and staff at the diabetes clinic at Aarhus University Hospital for allowing me to observe and raise questions during consultations. I also wish to thank a number of doctors across Denmark, who participated in interviews along the way. Your knowledge was much appreciated.

To the faculty at the Departments of Anthropology at both Aarhus University and Copenhagen University: I thank you all for sharing your ideas about my work at various seminars and conferences throughout the years. A special thank you to Susanne Højlund and Christian Suhr at Aarhus University for reading early chapter drafts of the doctoral thesis that eventually turned into this book and for giving me valuable feedback at a crucial time in the process. I further wish to thank the board that assessed my doctoral thesis and discussed it with me – Marcia Inhorn, Matthew Carey, and Maria Louw: our discussions qualified the arguments that I now get to present in this book. Thank you for your collegial support and encouragement to keep working with my material.

To my doctoral supervisors at Aarhus University: I thank, first of all, Anne Line Dalsgård for trusting in my intuition and encouraging me to creatively explore my analysis and writing; Mark Sedgwick for your insights on Cairo; and Nina Holm Vohnsen for raising questions that sharpened my arguments during the last months of writing my doctoral thesis. I also wish to thank Lila Abu-Lughod for hosting me at Columbia University in New York during the time of my doctoral research, and for encouraging me at the very beginning stages of my writing: you asked all the right questions.

To all the PhD students I shared time with at Aarhus University, I thank you for supporting me in ways surpassing the mere academic: Mette Lind Kusk, Thomas Mikkelsen, Laust Elbek, Annika Pohl Harrisson, Lars Hedegaard Williams, Abir Mohamad Ismail, and Theresa Ammann for coffees, talks and moral support throughout the process. To Maria Nielsen and Stina Møldrup Wolff for reading early drafts of my work and sharing experiences of motherhood while traveling the world and writing a doctoral thesis. To Mikel Venhovens and Søren Poulsen for reading early chapter drafts and laughing at my stories. And, finally, to Jonas Bach and Emilie Mortensen for reading and commenting on most parts of the doctoral thesis that has now turned into this book. I see your comments and questions reflected throughout all of the chapters. I am very grateful for the time and effort you both put into my work.

Thank you also to the anonymous reviewers who put effort into strengthening the arguments of the book. I appreciate your time and the work you put into helping me develop as a scholar.

I also wish to thank Routledge, specifically my editor Katherine Ong who initially welcomed my work and who has helped me carefully through the process.

To my family, especially my mother and Jørgen, I thank you for your unwavering support and for visiting me, Hussein, and Norr in Cairo and in New York. Aimee, I thank you for all of the time and support you put into reading my work and for your loving words. And finally, I thank Hussein, Norr, and Ronja –for your patience throughout the past years, and for sharing the adventure with me. I could not have done any of it without you. Thank you!

Note on Transliteration

I follow the standard system for transliteration of Arabic as outlined by the *International Journal of Middle East Studies* – with a few exceptions: in Cairo, the letter *jim*, or the "j" sound, is most often pronounced as a hard "g." When relevant I use a "g" instead of a "j" to reflect this. Furthermore, *qaf* is pronounced either as a "q" or as a glottal stop. I will transliterate it as a "q" throughout. I furthermore use the definite article of *il-* as opposed to *al-* when transliterating Egyptian colloquial expressions. In cases of certain names of people and places, I use *al-* (for example, President al-Sisi). In addition, I use the common English spelling of people and places whenever possible (for example, Mohamed as opposed to Moḥamad).

Prologue

Streaks of light are dancing on the office walls reflecting the numbers from a massive sign hanging on the outside walls of the building. The sign boasts the current population count of Egypt: 94,763,491 people. It is springtime in 2017, and my Egyptian friend Adam is accompanying me to the Department of Security Information at the Central Agency for Population Mobility and Statistics (CAPMAS) in Heliopolis, Cairo. I am trying to apply for a research permit. We are sitting in the office of the security officer who is also Head of the Department. He is sitting behind his desk, staring intensely at Adam and me. He is wearing a black suit and a big golden ring on his left little finger. It looks heavy and expensive. A TV is running in the background, airing news footage from a war-torn Yemen.

"I just want to make sure I am doing everything the right way, *'ayza imshī ṣaḥ*," I say to the officer, careful with my words, trying my best to sound polite.

He responds in Arabic, "You speak Arabic? *Batitkalimī 'arabī?*"

"I am learning, *bat'ālim*" I say, also in Arabic.

The officer nods. He shuffles through some papers before peering at me over the rim of his glasses. The conversation continues in Arabic.

"So, you want to talk to people you know already about their diabetes, and also to people *they* know about *their* diabetes?"

I nod.

"And after this, you will return to Denmark to study at a university there?"

I nod again.

He sits in silence for a while before asking, "You are not going to stop people in the streets, and ask them your questions?"

I shake my head. "No."

"And you do not work with the American Government?"

"No."

"The UN?"

"No."

He looks down at the table with his hands still folded. Finally, he says, "You don't need a permit."

I smile at the officer and then at Adam, surprised. Adam smiles back at me, I think with surprise as well. The officer finds a sticky note on his desk and writes his phone number and name on it before handing it to Adam. He looks at Adam intensely and says, "If anyone bothers her, they can call me directly."

Adam accepts the note and the security officer finally nods his head in the direction of the door, indicating that our conversation is over. I smile once more and thank him for his time.

"You welcome, you welcome," he says in English.

Adam and I quickly leave the office and continue down the hall. Adam has a wide grin on his face. I tell him that I did not know what to expect from our visit.

"Yeah, like everything with the government here," he says with a laugh. He continues, "I thought we would have to go to another office and then another office and then return ... and then not succeed. I guess he didn't find your research too important ... I mean ... sensitive ... or dangerous."

Questions

"Why are you here if you don't have diabetes?" Sherine, a young doctor, asks one of her patients in a diabetes clinic in Giza.

"You can't get diabetes because you are fat!" Ahmed, a young gardener, declares, while we both laugh at my assumption. "Enough! *Khalāṣ!*" he later exclaims, "You are going to give me diabetes with all these questions."

"Your aunt tells me the pill you give me is not good for me," a woman tells her son. "Well, that's not true," her son says.

"I stopped taking the pill. Someone told me the pills are bad for my kidneys," a patient later declares while the young man is at work as a doctor. "No, diabetes is bad for your kidneys, the pill will help you," he attempts to clarify.

A couple of women argue with a young pharmacist employed by a multinational medical company about the need to provide a prescription to retrieve an insulin pen, "I can get the pen today, and return tomorrow with *il-wara'a*, the paper," one of the women insists, while the pharmacist persistently turns her down.

A senior doctor raises her voice with patients in a waiting room, "Calm down!" she shouts.

"*Mā huwa maraḍ il-sukkar?* What is diabetes?" reads the front page of a brochure by a multinational medical company.

In the street in front of a public newspaper, a security officer angrily informs me, "You are not allowed to stand here! It's forbidden! What are you doing here?"

A friend asks, "*Kuntī khāʾyfa?* Were you scared?" later making sure, "You know the Arabic word *ḍaghṭ*, right?"

1 Introduction

This book deals with the topic of type-2 diabetes, more specifically with the tendency to raise questions in relation to existing knowledge of type-2 diabetes above accepting already-given answers. The book is set primarily in Cairo, Egypt, though it draws links to a diabetes clinic in Denmark, as well as to a multinational medical company and international diabetes research and guidelines. It tells a story of uncertainty, not only among people in Cairo, but also within medical research on type-2 diabetes more generally. The book raises the fundamental question of what uncertainty may generate in both bodies and societies at large.

My research is based on nine months of ethnographic fieldwork in Cairo, Egypt, and three months of ethnographic fieldwork in various locations in Denmark carried out during the years of 2015 and 2017. Throughout my research I focused primarily on people diagnosed with type-2 diabetes in the early stages of their condition. I show how many of the people I met in Cairo who were diagnosed with type-2 diabetes linked experiences of *ḍaghṭ*, translated as "pressure" or "stress," to the onset of their condition. Treatment thus came to revolve primarily around relieving those who were diagnosed with the condition of any *ḍaghṭ*, through resting and other means, contradicting the general advice of Egyptian doctors, for example, to stay physically active or lose weight.

The book explores the interactions of these two different understandings of type-2 diabetes: one related to the notion of *ḍaghṭ* and another related primarily to obesity. I explore how and why some of those who were diagnosed with type-2 diabetes in Cairo so persistently resisted the relation of type-2 diabetes to obesity, despite a constant foregrounding of this etiology among Egyptian healthcare personnel and authorities, as well as among multinational medical companies in the country. Drawing on existing social research from within Egypt (Schielke 2015; Hamdy 2012;

DOI: 10.4324/9781003327684-1

Mahmood 2012; Mitchell 2002; Malmström 2019) I argue that uncertainty historically has been used as a political tool in Egypt to maintain a firm grip on its population; however, throughout my research in Cairo, uncertainty was simultaneously invoked to resist this grip as well. Throughout the book I illustrate how uncertainty – manifested, for example, in the raising of questions – was used by people in Cairo to protect themselves, for example, from political, social, and medical harm. Paradoxically, this uncertainty was believed also by the people I worked with in Cairo to cause experiences of *ḍagḥṭ* and subsequently the condition of type-2 diabetes.

On an empirical level, this book tells the story of such experiences of *ḍagḥṭ* and how they manifested in inflation rates, rumors, conspiracies, paranoia, fear, corruption, love, and grief, as well as a range of other abstractions and specifics. As opposed to dealing with the management of type-2 diabetes through blood sugar measurements and regulated calorie intake, people in Cairo who were diagnosed with type-2 diabetes, and their family members, were instead concerned with how to manage factors such as shifting economies, rumors, and corruption in relation to their condition. They were asking questions such as: Why this sudden shortage of sugar and medicine? Is the doctor telling me the truth, or trying to profit from my suffering? Does the medicine work in the ways promised by my doctor? Will my brother's schizophrenia harm my father's diabetes? Will I be able to cultivate emotions of love upon marriage? What actually happened during recent years of political turmoil? "You are going to give me diabetes with all these questions," Ahmed, a young gardener, fittingly declared at one point during my research, partly joking, partly serious.

As a theoretical framework the book draws on recent discussions within the field of anthropology and science studies on topics of (un)certainty, doubt and (mis)trust (see, for example, Bubandt 2014; Carey 2017; Pelkmans 2013). This theoretical framework is drawn upon throughout the book to discuss how knowledge is produced and challenged; locally in Cairo, but also internationally within medical research. The overall aim of the book is to contribute to a better understanding of the growing global inequity of type-2 diabetes and its treatment (World Health Organization (WHO) 2016) by paying close attention to the questions and doubts raised by people in Cairo who are diagnosed with the condition. What can their doubts teach us about the condition of type-2 diabetes in Egypt specifically, but also in relation to a global medical scene?

"All of our doubts announce not the end of a story but the beginning of one," anthropologist Peter Metcalf once fittingly wrote (Metcalf 2003:16). This seems a suitable way to begin this book.

What We Know (About Diabetes and Other Things)

Even though diabetes is often coined an "epidemic" of our time (see, for example, Farag and Gaballa 2011; Zimmet 2017), it is widely recognized that features consistent with diabetes were accounted for in medical texts dating as far back as 1500 BC. It so happens that these early texts were ancient Egyptian, disclosing a condition in which patients suffered from excessive thirst and urination. Similar accounts can be found in other ancient medical literature originating from India and China. In later records from approximately 200 BC, a millennium after the early Egyptian writings, the condition of "diabetes" is mentioned more specifically. These records were written by Greek physicians trained at the Alexandrian school of medicine in Egypt.

The word "diabetes" was derived from the Ionic word "to pass" or "run through," referring to the quick and excessive passage of urine. At the time, the Greeks classified diabetes as a disease of the kidneys, having previously established the kidneys as the source of urine. Moving forward in time another two millennia to the AD 1600s, English physician Thomas Willis observed a sweet taste in the urine of those afflicted with diabetes. Willis observed that this sweetness appeared first in the blood and then in the urine, marking a paradigm shift in clinical descriptions of diabetes from one primarily focusing on urine to one primarily focusing on blood. Willis' observations gave diabetes its full name, "diabetes mellitus," "mellitus" meaning "honey-like" in Latin (for a thorough account of the above, see, for example, Eknoyan and Nagy 2005; Karamanou et al. 2016; Quianzon and Cheikh 2012; White 2014).

Although Willis related diabetes to a sweetness of the blood, the condition was still considered a disease of the kidneys. Around the same time of the discoveries of Willis, Swiss researchers experimented with removing the pancreas from dogs, observing that the dogs survived the removal. The pancreas was thus deemed a non-vital organ for many years to come. It was not until the 1800s that other European physicians confirmed the relation between the pancreas and diabetes, describing also the morphologic features of the pancreas (referred to as the pancreatic islands).

In 1916, English physiologist Edward Sharpey-Schafer suggested that these pancreatic islands produced a blood sugar regulating hormone necessary for the sugar to travel from the blood into the cells. Thus, he predicted the existence of insulin before its actual discovery. Sharpey-Schafer named the hormone "insulin" from the Latin word for "island" ("insula") (Eknoyan and Nagy 2005:226–7). In early 1922, a team of Canadian physicians and chemists managed to isolate the hormone and treat their first patient with animal-derived insulin (see, for example, Bliss 1993; Quianzon and Cheikh 2012; White 2014).

Up to this point, diabetes had been a fatal disease. The inability of the body to transfer sugar from the blood into the cells caused the body to burn fatty acids and produce acidic ketone bodies in the blood. This caused the patient to severely dehydrate, fall into a coma, and subsequently die of multiple organ failure (of course, this is still today a possible outcome of diabetes if the blood sugar level is not sufficiently regulated) (Chiasson et al. 2003). The insulin treatment carried out by the Canadian team in early 1922 turned out to be successful, and the team immediately undertook a joint venture with the American medical company Eli Lilly & Company (Lilly) to manufacture insulin for commercial use. Within only a year, insulin was being produced, sold, and used to treating diabetes in most Northern American and European countries. Diabetes was no longer necessarily a fatal disease. Part of the Canadian team who worked on isolating insulin were awarded the Nobel Prize in "Physiology or Medicine" in late 1923, marking one of the fastest recognitions of a medical discovery in the history of the Nobel Prize (Bliss 1993; Quianzon and Cheikh 2012; White 2014).

Lilly was granted a one-year exclusive license to produce insulin, but only in the US and Latin America. Shortly after the discovery of insulin, Danish physiologist August Krogh traveled to Canada to acquire the skills necessary to produce insulin. Krogh was granted a license to set up insulin production in Copenhagen, Denmark in early 1923, the first, in fact, in Europe. The production in Copenhagen laid the foundation stone of the medical company known today as Novo Nordisk (Novo) (Bliss 1993). To this day, Lilly and Novo dominate the global market of insulin, along with the French company Sanofi. As of 2016, Novo, Lilly, and Sanofi were also the three biggest manufacturers of the insulin available on the Egyptian market (Wirtz et al. 2016), with Novo covering approximately 80% of this market (according to conversations with employees at the regional office of Novo in Cairo). Since these early years of the 1920s, the production of insulin has evolved greatly, introducing multiple insulins to the market with variations in onset, peak, and duration. In the 1980s, genetically engineered insulin was launched, marking a paradigm shift from animal-derived insulin (primarily from pigs and cows) to what has since been coined "human insulin" (though synthetically produced in a laboratory) (Bliss 1993; White 2014). The first batch of insulin to enter the Egyptian market was exported from Novo's production in Copenhagen in 1934 (Mehling 2016).

Shortly after this first batch of insulin entered the Egyptian market, another discovery marked a paradigm shift in the history of diabetes. In 1936, English physician Harold Himsworth differentiated diabetes into two types: one that was receptive to insulin treatment, and one that was not. The latter type of patients, he argued, appeared to not lack insulin, but rather a sensitizing factor limiting the efficiency of insulin. Himsworth termed these two types of diabetes "insulin-sensitive" and "insulin-insensitive" diabetes (Himsworth 1936). These two types later evolved into type-1 and type-2 diabetes or juvenile-onset and adult-onset diabetes (Ferzacca 2012:412). Since Himsworth first presented his arguments, many other types of diabetes have been differentiated and acknowledged, long ago surpassing a mere division of an "insulin-sensitive" and "insulin-insensitive" diabetes, or a type-1 and a type-2 diabetes. As of 2014, The American Diabetes Association (ADA) has recognized four overall types of diabetes, including almost 60 subtypes (ADA 2014).

These many differentiations point to the fact that diabetes is defined by a common outcome, that is, a potentially elevated level of blood sugar, rather than a common physiological reason for this outcome. Thus, the diabetic body may completely lack the beta-cells needed in the pancreas to produce insulin, and therefore also lack completely insulin, but it may also produce insulin, yet, for one reason or another, this insulin is not sufficient or adequately efficient; something in the body may resist the action of insulin. Anthropologist Melanie Rock fittingly argues on the nature of diabetes, "A plethora of conditions that all share one feature – dangerously sweet blood – have been grouped together under the category of diabetes" (Rock 2003:137). As stated at the beginning of this introduction, this book focuses primarily on what is commonly referred to as type-2 diabetes. However, this category of diabetes has long ago surpassed Himsworth's definition of an "insulin-insensitive" type of diabetes. According to the ADA type-2 diabetes accounts for 90–95% of those with diabetes altogether, and encompasses individuals "who have insulin resistance and usually have relative (rather than absolute) insulin deficiency" (ADA 2014:S83).

Over the years, a broad range of medications have been developed to treat the different conditions of diabetes. In addition to the different types of insulin outlined above, as of 2014, there were ten different categories of diabetes medication (with many additional subcategories and "generations" of medicines) (White 2014). These medications vary greatly in mechanism and effect. Some, for example, work by improving the sensitivity of the body to insulin, others by reducing the glucose production in the liver. Some work by delaying gastric emptying, while others appear to lower the blood sugar level for reasons that are "not known" (see, for example, Quianzon and Cheikh 2012:3; or White 2014:85). In Egypt, as in Denmark, those who are diagnosed with diabetes, but who do not immediately require insulin treatment, are prescribed medication according to an algorithm stating the first choice of medicine, the second choice of medicine and so on (Nathan et al. 2006). The algorithm is based on currently available research indicating which pharmaceutical products have turned out to be the most beneficial to the most people. This approach is applied in diabetes treatment because it is often difficult, if not impossible, to differentiate exactly which subtype of diabetes the person is suffering from and thus what exactly should be targeted medically in the body. (During my research in Cairo, one doctor fittingly explained how much diabetes treatment was more of an "experiment" than an "exact science.")

In addition to medication, dieting plays a significant role in the history of diabetes treatment. Early ancient Egyptian medical texts outlined a treatment of diabetes that revolved around the intake of elderberry, fibers from the asit plant, milk, beer, cucumber flowers, and green dates (White 2014:82). Similarly, Willis, the English physician who observed the sweetness in the urine of those diagnosed with diabetes in the 1600s, outlined how a diet of vegetables, rice, milk, rhubarb, and cinnamon appeared to improve the condition of those diagnosed with diabetes (Karamanou et al. 2016:3–4). At the time of the discovery of insulin in 1922, dietary treatment of diabetics had evolved into the basic advice, "eat as little as possible" (Karamanou et al. 2016:6). This advice was given in an attempt to avoid high blood sugar levels following the intake of food, and the simultaneous inability of the body to assist the sugars in entering the cells.

The discovery of insulin and the development of other diabetes medications have not reduced the focus on dieting in relation to diabetes in the present, as those who depend on the injection of insulin still need to regulate their diet carefully. In practice, they are mimicking the balancing art of the pancreas, and thus need to coordinate rather precisely the dosage of insulin to their intake of food and physical exercise. Miscalculations may result in either a sudden drop or a sudden dramatic increase in the blood sugar level, with both scenarios being potentially lethal in an acute sense, but also over time because they increase the risk of other ailments such as cardiovascular disease, strokes, and organ failure (Kalra et al. 2013; Marcovecchio 2017). Those who have been diagnosed with diabetes, but who do produce insulin themselves, often benefit from losing weight and eating less. This is so as eating less reduces the amount of sugar that enters the body (and weight loss in general reduces the amount of sugar needed to sustain it). This in turn increases the likelihood that a natural production of insulin can keep up with the proper and timely transportation of sugar from the blood into the cells (Al-Goblan, Al-Alfi, and Muhammad 2014; Golay and Ybarra 2005).

This is where history catches up with the present and where the story starts to get blurry – for how obesity actually relates to diabetes as an overall disease category, and to the intake of certain foods and beverages, has been heavily disputed. Before exploring some of these disputes, let me first sum up what the above history of diabetes may teach us anthropologically about the notion of knowledge: It is evident in much of the literature drawn upon in the above that there is a certain vocabulary to knowledge. Knowledge may be discovered and developed, but it may also be discredited, disputed, and disclosed (it may even be predicted before its actual discovery, take for example Sharpey-Schafer's prediction of the existence of insulin). In the hindsight of history, knowledge may very well turn out to be misleading (such as the early experiments on dogs that deemed the pancreas a non-vital organ). On a similar note, knowledge may appear exhausted, and remain uncontested for millennia, while simultaneously consistently transforming over time (for example, from ascribing diabetes to a "condition of the kidneys" to a "condition of the pancreas," possibly resulting in "kidney disease" – or from the category of "diabetes" to "diabetes mellitus" to "type-1 and type-2 diabetes") (Eknoyan and Nagy 2005).

Anthropological literature has focused on knowledge as an object of research throughout its history, and major shifts in general anthropological debates are thus evident in a review of this literature. For example, literature published in the 1960s and 1970s focused primarily on the fundamental question of how knowledge acts on individuals through the shaping of policies and institutions (see, for example, Bourdieu 1990; Foucault 1970; and Foucault 1976 to list here only a few of the most groundbreaking works from this time). Literature published in the late 1980s and early 1990s rather focused on how individuals negotiate or move between different, sometimes contradicting, spheres of knowledge (see, for example, Abu-Lughod 1986; Barth 1993; Kleinman 1980).

The above historical account of diabetes tells us little about the ways in which specific knowledge of diabetes acted upon individuals throughout history, or how individuals negotiated between different spheres of knowledge – but it does tell us something about the epistemology of knowledge, evident also in the above well-reputed anthropological works: That knowledge may appear at one and the same time rigid and exhausted, as well as ever-changing and uncertain.

Recent science and technology studies within anthropology have explored how doubts and hesitations are fundamental to the generation of scientific knowledge, though often invisible from final research results (see, for example, Latour 1999; Latour 2010). Anthropologist Bruno Latour has famously illustrated how the scientific process in various academic fields is "made invisible by its own success." He elaborates, "When a machine runs efficiently, when a matter of fact is settled, one need focus only on its inputs and outputs and not on its internal complexity" (Latour 1999:304). Latour refers to the invisibility of such internal complexity – the unknowns in the process of what later becomes known as facts – as the "black box of scientific facts" (Latour 1999:23).

Early American pragmatists explored the relation between doubt and the formation of scientific knowledge already in the late 1800s and early 1900s. They particularly addressed ways of actively jumpstarting processes of doubt as a way to generate new ideas (see, for example, Dewey 1910; James 2000; Pierce 1998). In the words of Pierce, in order to generate new ideas, "There must be real and living doubt" (Pierce 1998:127). Dewey subsequently outlined the scientific method of "experimental thinking" as a way to incite such real and living doubt (Dewey 1910). This was, in fact, groundbreaking at the time, as most scientific research had consisted primarily of passive observations, not of dynamic experiments as such. This is evident also in the above historical account of diabetes, in which knowledge of diabetes was first based primarily on passive observations (for example, of the sweet smell and taste of urine), and later on actual experiments (for example, the removing and subsequent re-implanting of the pancreas in a dog).

In summary, knowledge may appear rigid and final (without a shadow of a doubt), but, in reality, it was doubt and uncertainty that led to its formation in the first place. Herein lies a fundamental paradox of knowledge; the mutual presence of doubt and belief. In the above historical account of diabetes, this paradox becomes increasingly visible as we reach the present. The unknown visibly starts to entangle with the known as, for example, known diabetes medication turns out to work in ways unknown even to those who discovered the medicine in the first place. From the outset of what we (apparently) know about diabetes today, we now take a leap into some of the unknowns and ask, what they all have to do with Egypt?

What We Don't Know

A good place to untangle some of the unknowns from the knowns of diabetes is in the realm of statistics. There is an overwhelming amount of statistics on diabetes: Prevalence rates of diabetes per number of people. Globally, regionally, and nationally. In rural areas and in urban areas. Differentiated by men and women. Differentiated by certain age groups. There are prevalence rates of diabetes adjusted to a common global age profile. Diabetes-related mortality rates. Comparisons of the prevalence of diabetes and obesity. Comparisons of the prevalence of diabetes and smoking. There are prevalence rates of undiagnosed diabetes. Comparisons of past and present. Estimates of a future. And there are statistics on healthcare expenditures dedicated to diabetes, compared across nations and regions, calculated in percentages and in "health dollars" (see, for example, IDF 2017; WHO 2016).

While these statistics supposedly mirror what is known about diabetes – the preface of a 2016 WHO report, for example, states that it "advances our understanding of trends in diabetes prevalence" (WHO 2016:4) – they simultaneously communicate a host of unknowns. Take some of the numbers and statements of this "Global Report on Diabetes" published by the WHO in 2016 as an example: The report is very blunt, "Being overweight or obese is strongly linked to diabetes" (WHO 2016:28). However, when examining the numbers in the report, the regions with the highest and lowest prevalence rates of diabetes as an overall category and overweight do not seem to match. The region of South-East Asia, for example, has the second highest estimated prevalence rate of diabetes, but the lowest estimated prevalence rate of overweight. The European region has the second highest estimated prevalence rate of overweight (close to The Americas that have the highest prevalence), but comes second to last in the estimated prevalence rate of diabetes (close to the region of Africa). Simultaneously, the report states that longer life expectancy and population growth constitute the main reasons for the increase of diabetes prevalence worldwide, rather than an increase in obesity and overweight as such (WHO 2016:25). Considering these statistics and statements, why does the report link diabetes so bluntly to overweight?

Biomedical research does outline the mechanism that relates overweight and obesity to type-2 diabetes rather clearly, so much so that the term "diabesity" is referenced in much medical research on the topic (see, for example, Farag and Gaballa 2011; Golay and Ybarra 2005; Zimmet 2017). The research outlines how obesity increases a variety of substances in the body that are involved in the development of insulin resistance, while also impairing the beta-cells used by the pancreas to produce insulin. In other words, obesity causes the individual to produce less insulin, and at the same time makes the body more resistant to it (Al-Goblan, Al-Alfi, and Muhammad 2014; Golay and Ybarra 2005). Both mechanisms alone, or combined, may result in a chronically elevated level of blood sugar, eventually meeting the requirements of a diabetes diagnosis.[1]

What causes obesity, on the other hand, is less clear. In 2016, a group of American researchers published an article in the Journal of the American Medical Association (JAMA) arguing that the American sugar industry paid and encouraged Harvard scientists in the 1960s to downplay and suppress scientific evidence that linked the intake of sugar to obesity and heart disease. Through historical documents, the article discusses how the Harvard scientists were paid to publish a literature review foregrounding the relation between the intake of fat, obesity, and heart disease, while simultaneously backgrounding the role of sugar (Kearns, Schmidt, and Glantz 2016). The literature review was published in 1967 (McGandy, Hegsted, and Stare 1967), and, according to the recent article cited above, it influenced US dietary policies in the years to come (specifically the heavy promotion of a low-fat diet).

The above medical article from 2016 triggered popular articles across European and North American media, questioning how the American sugar industry "sweetened" research in its favor (Howard 2016), altogether deeming it the grand "Sugar Conspiracy" (Leslie 2016). Since the publication of the 2016 article in JAMA, other researchers have questioned the conspiratorial elements of the story (see, for example, Johns and Oppenheimer 2018). Either way, the above 2016 article correlates with a recent shift in biomedical literature pointing to sugar rather than fat as the culprit in the high worldwide prevalence of overweight and obesity, correlating "diabesity" with an increase in the consumption of sugar as well.

Biomedical scientists are currently discussing which specific types and components of sugar are the actual triggers of obesity. The most recent literature tends to emphasize a correlation in the increase of "diabesity" with an increase in the consumption of soft drinks, pointing to a high intake of high fructose corn syrup as particularly critical (see, for example, Bray and Popkin 2014; Højlund 2014; Jeppesen 2014). Yet, this literature is not irrefutable: China, for example, appears among the countries with the lowest consumptions of sugars and fat per capita in the world (Ferdman 2015), yet holds an average prevalence rate of diabetes (IDF 2017). Another example stems from early 1990s Cuba when the country displayed the highest consumption of sugar per capita in the world, and yet experienced a decrease in obesity and diabetes (Højlund 2014).

I emphasize these unknowns and contradictions in biomedical understandings of obesity and type-2 diabetes here because they somehow manage to disappear and transform into known facts that guide type-2 diabetes treatment and prevention worldwide, particularly in relation to dietary advice on weight loss and weight control. Scientific facts, correlations, and causations of one set of local bodies manage to become matters-of-fact for a common global body: Obesity is the primary cause of type-2 diabetes. In other words, the complexity of the argument is black boxed, to draw on Latour's notion. Certain knowledge is foregrounded and established as fact, while other knowledge is backgrounded and, in many ways, left out of sight. Returning to the 2016 WHO report, other biomedical researchers have pointed to the lack of statistical correlation between obesity and diabetes in South-East Asia, discussing if this lack of correlation speaks primarily to other more critical risk factors of type-2 diabetes in the region, or if the definition of obesity should be adjusted to the South-East Asian body (Tabish 2007). In other words, should the definition of obesity be altered to a local body for the notion of "diabesity" to become evident in this part of the world as well?

"Correlations do not prove causation" (Bray and Popkin 2014:951), physician George Bray and economist and nutritionist Barry Popkin state in an article on the relation between sugar, obesity, and diabetes. As the 2016 WHO report shows us, neither are causations necessarily evident in statistical correlations. In other words, although biomedical literature tells us rather clearly that obesity may lead to type-2 diabetes, statistically, this causation is not evident in all parts of the world. Perhaps the statistics of the WHO report mirror the very nature of diabetes as an illness category that covers a great many physiological conditions, and equally is triggered by a great many different factors (and combinations of factors). "Diabesity" may be the most commonly mentioned etiology of diabetes, but risk factors such as age, genes, body-fat distribution, malnutrition at an early age and stress are also mentioned in the literature (see, for example, Mol 2008; Rock 2003; Zimmet 2017).

According to the International Diabetes Federation, as of 2017 Egypt ranked number eight among the countries with the highest number of people with diabetes in the world: 8.2 million Egyptians supposedly suffer from diabetes (IDF 2017:46). Comparing this number with the number of inhabitants in Egypt, this leaves Egypt with a prevalence rate of approximately 8.3%, which is, in fact, a little below the global average of 8.5% (as of 2014, WHO 2016:6). I could boost this number a little, for example, by giving you the age-adjusted prevalence rate of diabetes in Egypt, a much higher 17.3% (IDF 2017). The age-adjusted prevalence of diabetes is a fictitious number that indicates how many people would have diabetes if the life expectancy was the same (high) across the globe. In other words, if people lived longer and did not "succumb to death from other causes" (IDF 2017:72), how many people would suffer from diabetes in Egypt? 17.3%. I believe such a number is what anthropologist Anna Tsing describes as a standardization of difference, "As long as facts are apples and oranges, one cannot generalize across them; one must first see them as 'fruit' to make general claims" (Tsing 2011:89). Age-adjustments constitute the "fruit" in this context – an attempt to transform local bodies in their environments into a global common, while, at the same time, marking out significant differences between the two.

It should be evident by now that statistics and correlations in relation to type-2 diabetes can be easily adjusted (and particular numbers emphasized) to tell a specific story of a high, low, or average prevalence of type-2 diabetes, as well as of how obesity, fats, sugars, soft drinks, and other factors play a critical role in relation to the onset of the condition. In addition, it should be evident that knowledge of type-2 diabetes is constituted as much by unknowns as by knowns, even though the unknowns tend to disappear and transform into known treatment guidelines and common global facts about type-2 diabetes. In summary, the global diabetic body connects to local bodies in a mesh of ongoing biomedical research, statistics, treatments, and advice aimed at solving the "global burden" (WHO 2016:20) and "epidemic" (IDF 2017:7) of diabetes. But what does it mean to be a local body in a mesh of global connections and how do we approach such a study ethnographically? From an exploration of some of the knowns and unknowns that lay the grounds of this book, I now turn to outline the main research questions and theoretical approach of the coming chapters, in other words, what we would like to know or gain from this research.

What We Would Like to Know

To the best of my knowledge, the topic of type-2 diabetes had yet to be addressed anthropologically from within the region of the Middle East and North Africa throughout the years of my research and work with this book. Anthropologists Jessica Newman and Marcia Inhorn have previously pointed to chronic illnesses such as type-2 diabetes as an under-researched topic in the region (Newman and Inhorn 2015). In other words, I did not have a body of literature from within the region that I could draw inspiration from or use in the discussions of my findings. Perhaps for this reason, the analysis and findings presented throughout this book particularly revolve around the ways in which type-2 diabetes in an Egyptian context connects to the topic on a global scale.

Anthropologist Anna Tsing has unfolded how an ethnography of global connections may benefit from a focus on local "frictions" and "awkward engagements" (Tsing 2011:xi). She argues that intrinsic to globalism and capitalism is the notion of a free flow of goods, ideas, and money; yet, in reality, "motion does not proceed this way at all" (Tsing 2011:5). Rather, she argues, global movements are characterized by "friction." Tsing elaborates how, "Roads are a good image of conceptualizing how friction works: Roads create pathways that make motion easier and more efficient, but in doing so they limit where we go. The ease of travel they facilitate is also a structure of confinement" (Tsing 2011:6). In other words, friction is constituted by a simultaneous resistance and motion (just as knowledge is constituted by rigidness and evolvement). In this book, I draw on Tsing's arguments when raising the overall question of how the global epidemic of type-2 diabetes manifests in frictions and awkward engagements among local bodies in Cairo.

During my fieldwork, these frictions occurred among various groups of people, including those who were diagnosed with type-2 diabetes, their relatives, those at risk of developing the condition, doctors and pharmacists, and multinational medical companies and their employees, who promoted global products and certain medical ethics in the heart of Cairo.

I could specify the above research question, and ask also how global knowledge of the epidemic of type-2 diabetes interacted with other understandings of the condition among people in Cairo. Anthropologist Fredrik Barth has argued, on the reasons for exploring the notion of knowledge, "Knowledge provides people with materials for reflection and premises for action" (Barth 2002:1). In this book, I argue along similar lines to Barth, though I utilize the notion of knowledge as constituted equally by unresolved questions as by firm convictions. To doubt and to believe, simultaneously and separately, constitute ways of knowing.

Anthropologists Mathijs Pelkmans and Nils Bubandt, in particular, have turned to theorize on the notion of "doubt" in relation to various ethnographic fields. Whereas Pelkmans argues in his anthology on doubt that doubt tends to disappear and transform into belief "with the articulation of thought and the performance of action" (Pelkmans 2013:32), Bubandt rather argues from his work on witchcraft in Indonesia that doubt cannot always be sidelined or transformed into belief; at times it may simply be at rest (Bubandt 2014:6). Anthropologist Susan Whyte has previously argued along similar lines based on her work among people with HIV in Uganda that "uncertainty" does not necessarily transform into certainty by way of action and thought (Whyte 1997). Drawing on the works of Dewey (Dewey 1929), she argues, "Uncertainty is not to be denied, but acknowledged as a characteristic of both the experience of misfortune and the process of dealing with it" (Whyte 1997:19). Thus, Whyte holds that ethnographers ought not only to focus on experiences of uncertainty, but also on how people move ahead despite this uncertainty (Whyte 1997:226).

Resonating with the works of both Bubandt and Whyte, anthropologist Matthew Carey has recently argued from his work in Morocco that "mistrust" constitutes the primary scaffold of society in this particular ethnographic setting (Carey 2017). Carey thus opposes much sociological literature commonly outlining how "trust" (for example, in certain knowledge and people) constitutes a necessary social force without which societies would "disintegrate" (see, for example, Simmel 2004:178–9). "Mistrust," Carey holds, may similarly constitute such an integrating and necessary social force in certain empirical settings. In collaboration with anthropologist Morten Pedersen, Carey has further conceptualized how "infrastructures" of doubt and uncertainty may underpin societies in ways similar to the ways in which the social sciences have commonly outlined the workings of infrastructures of certainty and belief. More specifically Carey and Pedersen argue that uncertainty and doubt are generated and sustained in similar ways as certainty by the workings of "infrastructures," be they social, material, semiotic, or affective (Carey and Pedersen 2017:21).

The above discussions link to debates that run through the history of anthropology on "rational" versus "irrational" modes of thought and other distinctions such as "culture" versus "nature," "to know" versus "to believe," "modern" versus "nonmodern," "Us" versus "Them" (see, for example, Latour 1993; Said 1978). Latour famously attempted to dissolve these distinctions in his book first published in 1991, "We have never been modern," arguing that so-called "moderns" draw on their beliefs as much as "nonmoderns" – these beliefs are simply framed as "facts" (Latour 1993). Bubandt further sums up the arguments of Latour as follows: "Moderns need to believe in the belief of the other to maintain their own account of themselves as nonbelievers" (Bubandt 2014:15).

In the first part of this introduction, I outlined how facts are essentially established as certain knowledge is foregrounded, while certain knowledge is backgrounded. Some theories become truer and more accurate than others as uncertainties and inconsistencies disappear from immediate sight. Put differently, certain knowledge moves from complex spheres to simpler ones in the establishment of what becomes known as facts. Certain "facts" come to be deemed "rational," while others – and their promoters – are deemed "irrational." Relevant to the scope of this book: Considering the great many factors medically acknowledged as related to the onset of type-2 diabetes (see, for example, Mol 2008; Rock 2003; Zimmet 2017), why is the etiology of "diabesity" so persistently foregrounded over others?

In Cairo, this question was not only of relevance to me as an anthropologist, but also of relevance to the people who participated in my research. Questions such as: "Why is this information emphasized?" "What is left out of this story?" or "Who may benefit from this specific rendition of events and facts?" ran through many spheres of everyday life in Cairo, including those that related to type-2 diabetes and its treatment. In other words, backgrounded information did not disappear from sight to the people I worked with in Cairo; rather, the awareness of the possibility that information was being purposely left out of everything from medical advice to political decisions was ever-present among the people who participated in my research. "*Mish ʿarfa law ṣaḥ walla mish ṣaḥ*, I don't know if this is true or not true," people in Cairo persistently told me in relation to a range of issues, demonstrating the general sentiment that truth is always up for grabs, the intentions and workings of others intrinsic to what appears known about a given subject.

Several anthropologists and social scientists working in Egypt have touched on the topic of doubt and uncertainty in relation to various aspects of everyday life. These works include Schielke's work on conflicting ideals among Egyptian youth (Schielke 2009; Schielke 2015); Sherine Hamdy's work on the uncertainties of kidney patients with regard to, for example, religious ethics and the effects of the environment on the body (Hamdy 2008; Hamdy 2012); the work of Saba Mahmood (Mahmood 2012) and Charles Hirschkind (Hirschkind 2006) respectively in relation to religious faith and practice; Timothy Mitchell's work on the effects of foreign powers and so-called expertise on various aspects of social and political life in Egypt (Mitchell 2002); and more recently Mona El-Ghobashy (El-Ghobashy 2021) and Maria Frederika Malmström (Malmström 2019) on the political uncertainties in Egypt. In this book, I draw on the above works when presenting the overall argument that, in Cairo, structures of uncertainty underpinned society, encouraging and reinforcing a general tendency to raise questions, as opposed to merely accepting already-given answers.

Sociologist Jack Barbalet has previously argued that trust is "based on expectation, not deliberative calculation" (Barbalet 2009:378). In other words, trust points to future situations, "outcomes that have not occurred at the time of the choice to act or trust" (Barbalet 2009:378). Similarly, I argue from my fieldwork in Cairo that structures of uncertainty were facilitated by the expectations of others to act in certain (uncertain) ways. In other words, past experiences of political, social, and medical betrayal and misconduct formed people's future expectations of others to act in doubtful ways.

In the introduction to his anthology on doubt, Pelkmans fittingly argues how, "Doubt does not exclusively point to ontological and epistemological referents, to the questions 'what is?' and 'what is true?' Lived doubt points also (and sometimes more pressingly) to pragmatic referents, to the question 'what to do?'" (Pelkmans 2013:2). As outlined above, Whyte has similarly argued that ethnographers should not merely examine the ways in which people express their "uncertainties," but also the ways in which people move ahead despite these uncertainties (Whyte 1997:226). In similar ways, I ask from my research in Cairo how those diagnosed with type-2 diabetes explained and acted upon their condition in an everyday life constituted equally by uncertainty and doubt as by firm convictions. In other words, from questioning "What is true?" how did people come to form opinions of "What to do?"

Introducing Cairo

I first arrived in Cairo to conduct research for this study in May 2015. This was my second trip ever to Cairo as I had stayed in the city before, studying Arabic for six months in 2010. However, a very specific series of events set those two trips historically apart – the events of the Arab uprisings that had taken place not only in Egypt, but throughout the surrounding region in the winter and spring of 2011. Other anthropologists and social scientists have addressed the political despair within Egypt in the years up to 2011 (see, for example, Abu-Lughod and El-Mahdi 2011; Hamdy 2012; Prince 2014; Schielke 2015). Personally, I recall one of my language instructors in 2010 practicing with me slowly in Arabic, "Hosni Mubarak is the Egyptian president." After a pause, she added equally slowly, maybe in an attempt to have me recognize the future tense, "And when he dies, his son, Gamal Mubarak will be the Egyptian president." She immediately blushed in disbelief at what she had just indicated – that a rather corrupt president was in the process of passing on his presidential office to his son in an undemocratic way. Quickly, she added that the school did not allow her to discuss politics with her students; she apologized and moved on.

Just before I left Cairo in July 2010, a good friend of mine had shown me a group on Facebook called "*Kulina Khālid Sa'īd*, We Are All Khālid Sa'īd." The group administrators were spreading images and news about a young man, Khaled Said, who allegedly had been beaten to death by police officers in Alexandria in June 2010. The group was calling for rallies across the country in an attempt to raise a voice against an oppressive and violent police force. Fast-forward to early 2011, in the words of anthropologist Linda Herrera, the Facebook group "was on fire" (Herrera 2014:4). By the time of the initial demonstrations in Egypt in early 2011, the group had reached 390,000 members and received an average of 9 million hits a day (Herrera 2014:5).

Many factors have since been attributed to the successful mobilization of the Egyptian population in the years, months, and weeks up to and following the uprisings in early 2011, social media – including the Facebook group of *Kulina Khālid Sa'īd* – being just one (Herrera 2014). After the initial demonstrations on January

25, 2011 there were continuous demonstrations, sit-ins, and violent outbreaks between demonstrators, police, and military across Egypt. Chants such as "*Aysh, ḥurriya, 'idāla 'igtamā'ya*, Bread, freedom, social justice" became iconic of the events of these weeks. On February 11, 2011, 18 days after the initial demonstrations on January 25, Hosni Mubarak resigned as the Egyptian president after almost 30 years in office (El-Ghobashy 2021).

From the uprisings in 2011 to July 2015, two months into my research, I found myself in a different classroom, with a different language instructor, discussing a quote from a popular Egyptian book, *Taxi*, by Khaled Al-Khamissi (Al-Khamissi 2007). The book was published in 2007 during Mubarak's time and comments on social and political issues of the past and present. My language instructor and I were discussing a quote in which the time of President Hosni Mubarak was compared to the time of two previous presidents, Gamal Abdel Nasser and Anwar Sadat.[2] Translated from Arabic into English the quote goes, "The one, who did not get imprisoned during Nasser, will never go to prison. The one, who did not get rich during Sadat, will never get rich. The one, who will not become a beggar during Mubarak, will never beg" (Al-Khamissi 2007:84). I asked my language instructor how the quote would continue if we put in sitting President Abdel Fattah al-Sisi, elected in 2014 after the ousting of first-elected President Mohamed Morsi. He looked at me for a while and then proposed, "Maybe ... the one, who doesn't die during Sisi, will never die?"

I recall how we both laughed at his comment, yet the severity of it lingered. I found the comment a clever reference to the increasing state violence that I had both observed and been told about during these first two months of my fieldwork in 2015. In addition, the comment was a reference to a general sentiment among the Egyptians that I knew that President al-Sisi would surely manage to stay in office for many years to come and thus "outlive" everyone as a president. In 2017, when I returned for my second phase of fieldwork in Cairo, the country was undergoing a harsh economic crisis, partially due to the aftermath of the uprisings in 2011. In the spring of 2017, following several bombings targeting the Coptic community in Egypt, President al-Sisi declared a state of emergency in the country. He thus re-instated a political and legal scenario similar to the one that had allowed former President Mubarak to rule for almost 30 years. The political situation in Egypt at the time of my fieldwork affected both the everyday life of those who participated in my research, but also my own whereabouts in Cairo, the extent of my fieldwork stays in the country, and, importantly, it made the topic of uncertainty and its relation to type-2 diabetes the more prevalent (I have written about the methodological implications of conducting ethnographic fieldwork in Egypt during the years of 2015–17 elsewhere; see Thorsen 2020).

I have seen population counts of Cairo ranging from anywhere between 9.7 million (in the governorate of Cairo, CAPMAS.gov.eg 2018) to 18.5 million (as of 2008, Tignor 2011:302), depending on the source and demarcation. No matter which number is closer to reality, Cairo is, needless to say, a crowded and busy metropolis.[3] The city is cut through by the River Nile with several small islands along the way, some connected to the mainland by bridges, others accessible only by boat. To the east of the Nile, in the center of Cairo, one finds Tahrir Square, especially known outside of Egypt as a major rallying point during the Arab uprisings in 2011. To the west of the Nile, and a bit south along the river, one finds the Pyramids of Giza. Enclosing these two historical sights of Tahrir Square and the Giza Pyramids, one finds a countless number of different neighborhoods – many in which I conducted fieldwork for this book.

In other words, Cairo is not so much one single city, but rather a patchwork of neighborhoods and places each containing their own history and characteristics (see also Sims 2012). Perhaps for this reason, most of the Egyptians that I came to know during my fieldwork in Cairo expressed a strong relation to their specific neighborhoods. People were raising their own families in the same area (if not the same specific streets) where they had been born and raised themselves; neighbors appeared to know each other well and were often connected one way or another through marriages and kinship. Despite these strong local ties, almost everyone moved around the city on a regular basis to attend work or school, or to frequent certain hospitals, doctors' clinics, pharmacies, and so on. Similarly, I came to move around the city in what can be categorized as a "multi-sited" fieldwork (see, for example, Marcus 1995; and Marcus 2011 for more on the methodological discussions of "multi-sited" fieldwork).

Conducting Fieldwork in Cairo and Beyond

When I initially arrived in Cairo in 2015 to conduct the first phase of fieldwork for this book, I had arranged to stay with a family that I knew well from my previous stay in the city in 2010. The family lived in a tight-knit community on the northern outskirts of Cairo, and welcomed me into their home during the first month and a half of my fieldwork. I stayed with a young couple, Maha and Mustafa,[4] who had recently married and were now expecting their first child. Maha worked as an Arabic teacher in a public school down the street, and Mustafa worked with advertising at a public newspaper in downtown Cairo. Their parents were all retired, living on their pensions and savings. Most days were spent assisting Maha's mother-in-law and mother with chores and errands, as both were diagnosed with type-2 diabetes and rather ill from their condition. In addition, six of Maha's uncles and aunts (maternal and paternal) were diagnosed with type-2 diabetes, as was her maternal grandmother (and her late father). In other words, within Maha's family alone nine people were diagnosed with type-2 diabetes at the time of my fieldwork in 2015.

With the help of Maha and others in Cairo, I eventually established relations with four other families, who also had several family members diagnosed with type-2 diabetes. In the following chapters, I have chosen to focus on specific family members and their relations over others, as well as to link specific families primarily to specific chapters. I have chosen to do this to make the stories presented throughout the book more present to the reader. However, I wish to emphasize that a much larger number of people have contributed to the arguments presented throughout this book than what is explicitly visible on the coming pages. These include family members not cited or accounted for, as well as the literally hundreds of patients who passed through the various healthcare facilities that I worked with in Cairo, but who naturally did not all fit into the following chapters. I hope that the extent and depth of my fieldwork will be visible throughout the book, despite my zooming in on particular people and their stories.

The family members I have chosen to draw on in the following chapters are primarily Maha, Ahmed, Taher, Mai, and Mohamed; all were in their late 20s at the time of my fieldwork and all were children of parents diagnosed with type-2 diabetes. I made the choice to view this research on type-2 diabetes and its effects through the lens of these young relatives for two primary reasons.

First, the experience of being given a diagnosis of, for example, type-2 diabetes has often been discussed in research stemming from European and North American ethnographic settings as something similar to what sociologist Michael Bury has called a "biographical disruption" (Bury 1982); a life-altering experience marking a before and after the moment of diagnosis (see, for example, Ferzacca 2012 for a literature review). However, among those I worked with in Cairo who had been diagnosed with type-2 diabetes, the moment of diagnosis was not framed as a "biographical disruption" as such. Rather, the diagnosis seemed to be generally calmly accepted and often perceived as a natural part of aging. When writing this book, it thus became evident to me that narratives in Cairo of what leads up to a diagnosis of type-2 diabetes, and how it should subsequently be treated, were perhaps better told by those at risk: the young relatives shielding their parents and in-laws from experiences of *ḍaghṭ* related both to the onset and poor treatment of type-2 diabetes.

Second, much work and emotional labor was allocated to the younger family members in relation to diabetes treatment, including house chores, cooking, going to the market or the doctor's office, as well as, for example, keeping secrets from those diagnosed with type-2 diabetes as a way to protect them from potential distress. Treatment of type-2 diabetes thus appeared to revolve more so around the actions of young relatives than around the actions of those actually diagnosed with the condition. During my time with the families of Maha, Ahmed, Taher, Mai, Mohamed, and others I thus observed and participated in everyday life, assisting those young relatives with their endeavors.

The families and their members were employed in a broad range of fields. Some made a living by doing housework for other families; others by doing hard manual labor; others were employed in the public sector as teachers or officials; others worked privately as translators and tour guides; and some no longer worked, but lived primarily on their pensions. Most of the members of the younger generation held university degrees from one of the public universities in town.

Anthropologist Samuli Schielke has argued on the classification of social classes in Egypt that, "Being middle class has become an ideal of social normality. People ranging from very poor to very wealthy have come to see themselves as middle class" (Schielke 2015:111). I find it difficult to classify the families that I worked with in Cairo as other than "middle class," although the families differed greatly with regard to income and financial abilities. None of the families belonged to what I would define as the upper class, that is, families who usually reside in the gated communities in the desert or in the neighborhoods of Zamalek or Maadi. Similarly, none of the families belonged to what I would define as the lower class, that is, families who struggle to make a living.

During my first months of fieldwork in Cairo, I reached out to the regional office of Novo, the multinational medical company that was the first company to produce insulin in Europe, and the first to introduce insulin to the Egyptian market, upon realizing that the company was heavily engaged in a number of public outpatient clinics for diabetics across Egypt. Novo quickly agreed to assist me with my research, both in the form of interviews with employees and by establishing contact with two different types of diabetes clinics in Cairo. One of these clinics was a so-called Novo Care Center situated in the neighborhood of Dokki, owned and run by Novo themselves. In this center, people could retrieve the NovoPen (a device used to inject insulin) for free on referral from a doctor. The other clinic was a public outpatient clinic for diabetics in the neighborhood of Giza in which Novo cooperated with the Egyptian Ministry of Health, partially by financing the facilities in the clinic, and partially by attempting to gather patient data electronically. I will elaborate on the work in both of these clinics in Chapters 2 and 6.

With the assistance of my network in Cairo, I was gradually introduced to other people and institutions who were working directly or peripherally with people with type-2 diabetes. Thus, I also came to conduct parts of my fieldwork at a general practitioner's office in downtown Cairo, focusing especially on the initial diagnostic stages of type-2 diabetes; in an emergency room and intensive care unit at one of the university hospitals in Cairo, gaining insights into the possible acute dangers of type-2 diabetes; and in a privately owned pharmacy in Agouza, focusing particularly on those with type-2 diabetes who consulted the pharmacist for blood sugar measurements, injections of insulin, and general advice. In summary, my fieldwork was formed largely by way of what is commonly known within ethnographic methodology as the "snowball effect" (see, for example, Noy 2008), in many ways coincidental and based on the relations and assistance of people I already knew. In addition to the above, my fieldwork was qualified by meetings with strangers such as taxi drivers, fellow passengers on the metro, or shop owners willing to engage in conversations in passing.

In Cairo, I drew primarily on the ethnographic methods of participant observation and semi-structured interviews. The participant observations extended across the spectrum of primarily participating in activities, rather than merely observing them, to primarily observing activities, rather than participating actively in them (see, for example, Rabinow 1977; Robben and Sluka 2007; Spradley 1980). For example, when visiting the families I was working with the closest, I often participated in daily activities to an extent that made it difficult for me to take written notes of these events as they were occurring. In these cases, I would often spend my nights writing field notes from my memory alone, or based on a few notes, words, or quotes that I had scribbled down in a hurry. When visiting clinics and doctors' offices, on the other hand, I usually participated very little in the consultations, and thus had time to take extensive notes that would later assist me in a write-up of my field notes.

In addition to participant observation, I conducted a total of 16 semi-structured interviews (see, for example, Kvale and Brinkmann 2009) with family members diagnosed with type-2 diabetes in Cairo and 33 semi-structured interviews with healthcare personnel across various healthcare facilities. Most participant observations and interviews took place in Arabic, though I occasionally had conversations with younger people in English, or a mix of English and Arabic. Conversations and quotes have been translated from Arabic to English throughout the book unless otherwise stated. I have added transliterations wherever I have thought it relevant in relation to the context.

In addition to gathering my empirical data from participant observations, interviews, and casual conversations with strangers, I also gathered information from Egyptian media (newspapers, magazines, and TV), and from social media. This all added to my general understanding of the political and social context in Egypt at the time of my research. In addition to the above, my fieldwork in Cairo reached beyond my actual physical presence in the city, as I stayed in close contact with many of the people I had been working with when I was outside the country. I also followed the news and social media closely throughout my years of research, which continuously fed into my analysis and the writing of this book.

Before moving forward, I would like to discuss the ethics and consent of my research. It was often difficult for me to take notes during my visits with the families I was working with. Yet, I always carried a notebook with me, leaving it out on counters and tables, inviting people to scribble down notes, words, quotes, or questions, for example, whenever I needed assistance with the exact phrasing in Arabic, or if I was occupied physically elsewhere (with children, cooking, or something similar). This worked as a constant reminder to myself and others that our (sometimes close) relations also had a professional dimension. Maha, whom I stayed with during the first month and a half of my fieldwork in 2015, often read my field notes, and clarified any questions that I might have in relation to the past day's events.

In the case of intimate situations that did not relate directly to the topic of type-2 diabetes, but still came to matter in relation to this book, I reached out to the people in question to retrieve confirmation that I could use their story. This was the case particularly with the girls who form the basis of my analysis in Chapter 5. On a more formal note, I was in contact with Egyptian authorities at both the American University of Cairo and at the CAPMAS office respectively in 2015 and later in 2017 inquiring about the need to apply for a research permit. I was told both in 2015 and in 2017 that I did not need formal permission as such for my type of research. Working in clinics and hospitals across Cairo, I was granted permission by the directors or owners of these locations directly. Patients were informed about the purpose of my presence during consultations, generally welcoming me to Egypt and also my research on diabetes.

Both my fieldwork stays in Cairo in 2015 and in 2017 were cut short due the insecurity of the political situation in Egypt at the time. In 2017, I was beginning to focus on the ways in which type-2 diabetes travels globally (in forms of research, treatment, equipment, medicine, data, and so on), and how it manifests locally, in the present case, in Cairo. I discovered that one of the outpatient clinics that I was working with in Cairo, through Novo, had connections with an outpatient clinic for diabetics in Aarhus, Denmark. I therefore decided to conduct fieldwork in Denmark as well. I spent approximately three months primarily in the fall of 2017 conducting participant observation studies at the outpatient clinic for diabetics in Aarhus and performing a total of 14 semi-structured interviews with endocrinologists and other healthcare personnel across the country. While the data gathered from my fieldwork in Denmark is not explicitly visible in this book apart from one vignette in Chapter 6, it still fed into the formation of the book in many ways, including in relation to the overall frame of (un)certainty and doubt, as well as in relation to qualifying my general understanding of type-2 diabetes and current diabetes research (and debates).

Outline of the Chapters

In Chapter 2, Laughter, I outline how sentiments of uncertainty carry a long history in Egypt as a political tool used to control the population; however, I also illustrate how uncertainty was invoked by the general population in Cairo during my years of research to resist and protect themselves from political, social, and medical harm. I argue that humor and laughter especially provided the people I worked with in Cairo with a common space of communication – without succumbing to the certainty of specific narratives or so-called facts. Humor and laughter were thus drawn upon in many spheres of everyday life, including during medical consultations.

In Chapter 3, Food, I outline how experiences of *ḍaghṭ* were most commonly related to the onset of type-2 diabetes among those I worked with in Cairo who were diagnosed with the condition. I show how this etiology of *ḍaghṭ* contrasted one of "diabesity" emphasized by doctors and other healthcare personnel in Cairo. I illustrate the difference between the two by focusing on the topic of food specifically. I show how the intake of food was related to type-2 diabetes by those in Cairo who were diagnosed with the condition; not in relation to the number of calories or composition of nutrients consumed, but in relation to political and environmental factors affecting, for example, the price, availability, and quality of food. Overall, I argue that the people I worked with in Cairo who were diagnosed with type-2 diabetes did not relate their condition to neoliberal ideas of individual "lifestyle choices," but rather to factors in their surroundings.

In Chapter 4, Drugs, I explore the ways in which people in Cairo persistently raised questions and concerns over the intake of pharmaceuticals, acutely aware that pharmaceutical drugs are matters affected by the environments they are born into and travel through. Pharmaceutical drugs were thus not merely considered potential treatments among the people that I worked with in Cairo, but also as potential causes of illness; the uncertainty of, for example, availability, prices, contaminations, and the like causing experiences of *ḍaghṭ*, and potentially the onset of type-2 diabetes. Overall, I use the questions and concerns raised by people in Cairo to discuss the ways in which the pharmaceutical industry contributes to defining the problem of type-2 diabetes as one primarily of individual bodies and behavior. I argue that the ability to medicate individual bodies contributes to a backgrounding of other factors known biomedically to impact the onset and condition of type-2 diabetes, such as political and social structures.

In Chapter 5, Care, I illustrate how the etiology of *ḍaghṭ* caused the families that I worked with in Cairo to treat type-2 diabetes primarily by relieving those who were diagnosed with the condition of situations potentially invoking experiences of *ḍaghṭ*. However, I argue, relieving family members of such experiences did not simply make the *ḍaghṭ* go away; rather, pressures of everyday life carried the risk of shifting from the person diagnosed with type-2 diabetes to the relatives involved in their care, essentially placing those relatives at risk of developing type-2 diabetes themselves. Overall, I discuss the ways in which type-2 diabetes, a condition commonly framed within biomedical research as a non-communicable illness, carried risks of transmission within the family households that I worked with in Cairo.

In Chapter 6, Novo, I turn to address the role of the multinational pharmaceutical company Novo Nordisk in relation to diabetes care in Cairo. I specifically discuss the attempts of Novo to affect diabetes care in specific ways through the establishment of their own Novo Care Centers, but also through their engagement with the public healthcare sector. I explore how Novo appropriated specific understandings of certainty and objectivity; certainty in etiologies and treatments, but also, for example, in legal documents and what they perceived as proper medical ethics. However, I argue, such certainty, contrary to its intentions, came to pose a barrier to diabetes treatment to people in Cairo in different ways.

In Chapter 7, Final Notes, I turn to conclude on the arguments of the book. I suggest that digging into stories of uncertainty as presented throughout the chapters of this book could be one place to begin to improve type-2 diabetes care in Egypt – by acknowledging the experiences of those diagnosed with the condition, not merely in order to tap into the understanding of the local, but as a way to recognize that the high prevalence of type-2 diabetes in Egypt, and in this region at large, relate to much more complex issues than merely an excess consumption of food and calories.

Notes

1 The WHO and other associations have defined the range of a normal blood sugar level and an elevated blood sugar level respectively, categorizing those with a prolonged elevated blood sugar level as diabetic. Most countries (including Egypt) follow the recommendations and guidelines set forth by the WHO as to the specifics of these levels.

2 Nasser was the president of Egypt in the years 1954–1970, Sadat in the following years, 1970–1981.

3 The total population of Egypt is approximately 97.8 million as of November 2018 according to Egypt's Central Agency for Public Mobilization and Statistics. The majority of people live in and around Cairo and Alexandria (the second largest city in Egypt, situated in the north of the country on the Mediterranean shore).

4 All names of people involved in my fieldwork are pseudonyms. Most places have been anonymized except from the Novo Care Center in Dokki, the outpatient clinic in Giza and the outpatient clinic in Aarhus. Those clinics all carried unique characteristics and relations essential as part of the context of the analysis that rendered them impossible to anonymize. The same applied to Novo Nordisk. Both the clinics and Novo Nordisk were aware of their unique positions. Consent not to

anonymize the specific clinics and Novo Nordisk as a company was retrieved at the beginning of my study from the regional director of Novo Nordisk in Cairo. All personnel and patients within these facilities have, however, been anonymized.

References

Abu-Lughod, Lila. 1986. *Veiled Sentiments: Honor and Poetry in a Bedouin Society*. University of California Press.
Abu-Lughod, Lila, and Rabab El-Mahdi. 2011. Beyond the "Woman Question" in the Egyptian Revolution. *Feminist Studies* 37(3): 683–691.
ADA. 2014. Diagnosis and Classification of Diabetes Mellitus. *Diabetes Care* 37(1): S81–S90.
Al-Goblan, Abdullah S., Mohammed A. Al-Alfi, and Z. Muhammad. 2014. Mechanism Linking Diabetes Mellitus and Obesity. *Diabetes, Metabolic Syndrome and Obesity: Targets and Therapy* 7: 587–591.
Al-Khamissi, Khaled. 2007. *Taxi*. Dar al-shorouq.
Barbalet, Jack. 2009. A Characterization of Trust, and Its Consequences. *Theory and Society* 38(4): 367–382.
Barth, Fredrik. 1993. *Balinese Worlds*. University of Chicago Press.
Barth, Fredrik. 2002. An Anthropology of Knowledge. *Current Anthropology* 43(1): 1–18.
Bliss, Michael. 1993. The History of Insulin. *Diabetes Care* 16(3): 4–7.
Bourdieu, Pierre. 1990. *The Logic of Practice*. Stanford University Press.
Bray, George A., and Barry M. Popkin. 2014. Dietary Sugar and Body Weight: Have We Reached a Crisis in the Epidemic of Obesity and Diabetes? *Health Be Damned! Pour on the Sugar*. *Diabetes Care* 37(4): 950–956.
Bubandt, Nils. 2014. *The Empty Seashell: Witchcraft and Doubt on an Indonesian Island*. Cornell University Press.
Bury, Michael. 1982. Chronic Illness as Biographical Disruption. *Sociology of Health & Illness* 4(2): 167–182.
CAPMAS.gov.eg. 2018. *Census*. Egypt: Central Agency for Public Mobilization and Statistics.
Carey, Matthew. 2017. *Mistrust: An Ethnographic Theory*. Hau Books.
Carey, Matthew, and Morten Axel Pedersen. 2017. Introduction: Infrastructures of Certainty and Doubt. *The Cambridge Journal of Anthropology* 35(2): 18–29.
Chiasson, Jean-Louis, Nahla Aris-Jilwan, Raphaël Bélanger, et al. 2003. Diagnosis and Treatment of Diabetic Ketoacidosis and the Hyperglycemic Hyperosmolar State. *Canadian Medical Association Journal* 168(7): 859–866.
Dewey, John. 1910. *How We Think*. Dover Publications.
Dewey, John. 1929. *The Quest for Certainty*. Capricorn Books.
Eknoyan, Garabed, and Judit Nagy. 2005. A History of Diabetes Mellitus or How a Disease of the Kidneys Evolved into a Kidney Disease. *Advances in Chronic Kidney Disease* 12(2): 223–229.

El-Ghobashy, Mona. 2021. *Bread and Freedom: Egypt's Revolutionary Situation*. Stanford University Press.

Farag, Youssef M. K., and Mahmoud R. Gaballa. 2011. Diabesity: An Overview of a Rising Epidemic. *Nephrology Dialysis Transplantation* 26(1): 28–35.

Ferdman, Roberto A. 2015. Where People around the World Eat the Most Sugar and Fat. February 5 2015. The Washington Post. www.washingtonpost.com/news/wonk/wp/2015/02/05/where-people-around-the-world-eat-the-most-sugar-and-fat/?noredirect=on&utm_term=.ea32f39035e1.

Ferzacca, Steve. 2012. Diabetes and Culture. *Annual Review of Anthropology* 41: 411–426.

Foucault, Michel. 1970. *The Order of Things: An Archeology of the Human Sciences*. Pantheon Books.

Foucault, Michel. 1976. *The Birth of the Clinic: An Archeology of Medical Perception*. Tavistock Publications.

Golay, Alain, and Juan Ybarra. 2005. Link between Obesity and Type 2 Diabetes. *Best Practice & Research. Clinical Endocrinology & Metabolism* 19(4): 649–663.

Hamdy, Sherine F. 2008. When the State and Your Kidneys Fail: Political Etiologies in an Egyptian Dialysis Ward. *American Ethnologist* 35(4): 553–569.

Hamdy, Sherine F. 2012. *Our Bodies Belong to God: Organ Transplants, Islam, and the Struggle for Human Dignity in Egypt*. University of California Press.

Herrera, Linda. 2014. *Revolution in the Age of Social Media: The Egyptian Popular Insurrection and the Internet*. Verso Books.

Himsworth, Harold P. 1936. Diabetes Mellitus: Its Differentiation into Insulin-Sensitive and Insulin-Insensitive Types. *The Lancet* 227(5864): 127–130.

Hirschkind, Charles. 2006. *The Ethical Soundscape: Cassette Sermons and Islamic Counterpublics*. Columbia University Press.

Højlund, Susanne. 2014. Tasting Time: The Meaning of Sugar in Cuba. Contextualizing the Taste of Sweetness. *In Sugar and Modernity in Latin America: Interdisciplinary Perspectives*. Vinicius de Carvalho, Susanne Højlund, Per Bendix Jeppesen, and Karen-Margrethe Simonsen, eds. Pp. 73–93. Aarhus University Press.

Howard, Jacqueline. 2016. How the Sugar Industry Sweetened Research in Its Favor. September 12 2016. CNN. https://edition.cnn.com/2016/09/12/health/sugar-industry-heart-disease-research/index.html.

IDF. 2017. *IDF Diabetes Atlas*. Eighth Edition 2017. www.diabetesatlas.org/.

James, William. 2000. *Pragmatism and Other Writings*. Penguin Publishing Group.

Jeppesen, Per Bendix. 2014. Is There a Correlation between High Sugar Consumption and the Increase in Health Problems in Latin America? *In*

Sugar and Modernity in Latin America: Interdisciplinary Perspectives. Vinicius de Carvalho, Susanne Højlund, Per Bendix Jeppesen, and Karen-Margrethe Simonsen, eds. Pp. 25–55. Aarhus University Press.

Johns, David Merritt, and Gerald M. Oppenheimer. 2018. Was There Ever Really a "Sugar Conspiracy"? *Science* 359(6377): 747–750.

Kalra, Sanjay, Jagat Jyoti Mukherjee, Subramanium Venkataraman, et al. 2013. Hypoglycemia: The Neglected Complication. *Indian Journal of Endocrinology and Metabolism* 17(5): 819.

Karamanou, M., A. Protogerou, G. Tsoucalas, G. Androutsos, and E. Poulakou-Rebelakou. 2016. Milestones in the History of Diabetes Mellitus: The Main Contributors. *World Journal of Diabetes* 7(1): 1–7.

Kearns, C. E., L. A. Schmidt, and S. A. Glantz. 2016. Sugar Industry and Coronary Heart Disease Research: A Historical Analysis of Internal Industry Documents. *JAMA* 176(11): 1680–1685.

Kleinman, Arthur. 1980. *Patients and Healers in the Context of Culture: An Exploration of the Borderland between Anthropology, Medicine, and Psychiatry*. University of California Press.

Kvale, Steinar, and Svend Brinkmann. 2009. *InterViews: Learning the Craft of Qualitative Research Interviewing*. SAGE Publications.

Latour, Bruno. 1993 [1991]. *We Have Never Been Modern*. Harvard University Press.

Latour, Bruno. 1999. *Pandora's Hope: Essays on the Reality of Science Studies*. Harvard University Press.

Latour, Bruno. 2010. *The Making of Law: An Ethnography of the Conseil d'État*. Polity Press.

Leslie, Ian. 2016. The Sugar Conspiracy. April 7, 2016. The Guardian. www.theguardian.com/society/2016/apr/07/the-sugar-conspiracy-robert-lustig-john-yudkin.

Mahmood, Saba. 2012. *Politics of Piety: The Islamic Revival and the Feminist Subject*. Princeton University Press.

Malmström, Maria Frederika. 2019. *The Streets Are Talking to Me: Affective Fragments in Sisi's Egypt*. University of California Press.

Marcovecchio, Loredana. 2017. Complications of Acute and Chronic Hyperglycaemia. *US Endocrinology* 13(1): 17–21.

Marcus, George E. 1995. Ethnography in/of the World System: The Emergence of Multi-Sited Ethnography. *Annual Review of Anthropology* 24(1): 95–117.

Marcus, George E. 2011. Multi-Sited Ethnography: Five or Six Things I Know about It Now. *In Multi-Sited Ethnography: Problems and Possibilities in the Translocation of Research Methods*. S. Coleman, and P. V. Hellermann, eds. Pp. 24–40. Routledge.

McGandy, Robert B., D. M. Hegsted, and F. J. Stare. 1967. Dietary Fats, Carbohydrates and Atherosclerotic Vascular Disease. *New England Journal of Medicine* 277(4): 186–192.

Mehling, Nicholas. 2016. In Egypt, Novo Nordisk Leads the Fight in the Global War on Diabetes. May 30 2016. Daily News Egypt. https://

dailynewsegypt.com/2016/05/30/egypt-novo-nordisk-leads-fight-global-war-diabetes/.
Metcalf, Peter. 2003. *They Lie, We Lie: Getting on with Anthropology*. Routledge.
Mitchell, Timothy. 2002. *Rule of Experts: Egypt, Techno-Politics, Modernity*. University of California Press.
Mol, Annemarie. 2008. *The Logic of Care: Health and the Problem of Patient Choice*. Routledge.
Nathan, David M., John B. Buse, Mayer B. Davidson, et al. 2006. Management of Hyperglycemia in Type 2 Diabetes: A Consensus Algorithm for the Initiation and Adjustment of Therapy: A Consensus Statement from the American Diabetes Association and the European Association for the Study of Diabetes. *Diabetes Care* 29(8): 1963–1972.
Newman, Jessica, and Marcia C. Inhorn. 2015. Medical Anthropology in the Middle East and North Africa. *In A Companion to the Anthropology of the Middle East*. Soraya Altorki, ed. Pp. 205–232. John Wiley & Sons.
Noy, Chaim. 2008. Sampling Knowledge: The Hermeneutics of Snowball Sampling in Qualitative Research. *International Journal of Social Research Methodology* 11(4): 327–344.
Pelkmans, Mathijs. 2013. *Ethnographies of Doubt: Faith and Uncertainty in Contemporary Societies*. I. B. Tauris.
Pierce, Charles S. 1998. *The Essential Writings*. Prometheus Books.
Prince, Mona. 2014. *Revolution Is My Name: An Egyptian Woman's Diary from Eighteen Days in Tahrir*. The American University in Cairo Press.
Quianzon, Celeste, and Issam Cheikh. 2012. History of Current Non-Insulin Medications for Diabetes Mellitus. *Journal of Community Hospital Internal Medicine Perspectives* 2(3): 19081.
Rabinow, Paul. 1977. *Reflections on Fieldwork in Morocco*. University of California Press.
Robben, Antonius, and Jeffrey A. Sluka. 2007. *Ethnographic Fieldwork: An Anthropological Reader*. Blackwell Publishing.
Rock, Melanie. 2003. Sweet Blood and Social Suffering: Rethinking Cause-Effect Relationships in Diabetes, Distress, and Duress. *Medical Anthropology* 22(2): 131–174.
Said, Edward W. 1978. *Orientalism*. Penguin.
Schielke, Samuli J. 2009. Ambivalent Commitments: Troubles of Morality, Religiosity and Aspiration among Young Egyptians. *Journal of Religion in Africa* 39(2): 158–185.
Schielke, Samuli J. 2015. *Egypt in the Future Tense: Hope, Frustration, and Ambivalence before and after 2011*. Indiana University Press.
Simmel, Georg. 2004. *The Philosophy of Money*. Routledge.
Sims, David. 2012. *Understanding Cairo: The Logic of a City out of Control*. The American University in Cairo Press.
Spradley, James P. 1980. *Participant Observation*. Wadsworth Thomson Learning.

Tabish, Syed Amin. 2007. Is Diabetes Becoming the Biggest Epidemic of the Twenty-First Century? *International Journal of Health Sciences* 1(2): 5–8.

Thorsen, Mille K. 2020. Risky Notes: Reading Tense Situations in Cairo in 2015. *In Anthropology Inside Out: Fieldworkers Taking Note*. A. Andersen, L. Dalsgård, M. L. Kusk, et al., eds. Pp. 135–150. Sean Kingston Publishing.

Tignor, Robert L. 2011. *Egypt: A Short History*. Princeton University Press.

Tsing, Anna L. 2011. *Friction: An Ethnography of Global Connection*. Princeton University Press.

White, John R. 2014. A Brief History of the Development of Diabetes Medications. *Diabetes Spectrum* 27(2): 82–86.

WHO. 2016. *Global Report on Diabetes*. World Health Organization.

Whyte, Susan R. 1997. *Questioning Misfortune: The Pragmatics of Uncertainty in Eastern Uganda*. Cambridge University Press.

Wirtz, V., R. Knox, C. Cao, et al. 2016. *Insulin Market Profile*. April 2016. Health Action International.

Zimmet, Paul Z. 2017. Diabetes and Its Drivers: The Largest Epidemic in Human History? *Clinical Diabetes and Endocrinology* 3(1): 1–8.

2 Laughter

Anthropologist Talal Asad has outlined how Egyptian politicians, authorities, and media frequently warn the Egyptian population of so-called infiltrators; individuals believed to be planting or attempting to control public narratives with the aim of harming the Egyptian national state. Such infiltrators are often portrayed as affiliated with foreign national states or entities such as, for example, Israel or Iran, or multinational companies more generally, but they may also be portrayed as common thugs or remnants of the regime originating from within Egypt. According to Asad, attempts by both the Egyptian state and those so-called infiltrators to control public narratives in relation to a range of issues in Egypt have resulted in a high level of skepticism within the Egyptian population. This skepticism manifests in the ways many Egyptians persistently question, for example, participations and motives in violent outbreaks, election outcomes, and the like, of so-called foreign and local infiltrators, but also of Egyptian politicians and authorities: Who is telling the story and what do they have to gain? (Asad 2012).

In August 2014, Egyptian cartoonist Andeel published a satirical cartoon on the independent Egyptian-run online media Madamasr.com entitled, "One thing at a time." The cartoon depicts what appears to be President al-Sisi (although he is not named directly) sitting in his office, as a white male official walks in and asks, "Sir, sir, what are we going to do with the trash, the traffic, electricity, hospitals, security, wages, job opportunities and the future? What will we do with all the ignorance!!!" President al-Sisi responds, "...increase the ignorance." To me this cartoon illustrates the theoretical arguments of Asad rather well, fundamentally, because the narrative and the villain of the story are not clear: the joke is on whom?

The cartoon appears to be addressing the general sentiment among many Egyptians of being kept in the dark on important

DOI: 10.4324/9781003327684-2

political matters, or that attempts are being made to fool them into a certain understanding of reality; the idea that "increasing the ignorance" within the Egyptian population would allow al-Sisi to stay in office and promote his own needs over the needs of the general population.

However, the cartoon also communicates another possible story of a white official rushing to the office of what appears to be President al-Sisi raising social issues that can essentially be traced back to colonial interference in the country (see, for example, Inhorn 1994 and Mitchell 2002 for discussions on the impact of colonialism on Egyptian society). In addition, this official is given a response that mimics a prejudiced idea of a supposedly "ignorant" Egyptian population; an idea I encountered throughout my research among Egyptian healthcare personnel, as well as among multinational medical companies and their local and international employees, in their recounts of Egyptian patients not following medical advice due to their "ignorance." In other words, the narrative of the cartoon may also be perceived as a comment on the continuous interferences and impact of foreign powers and ideas in the country – manifested, for example, in the presence of international organizations and companies and their attempts to influence Egyptian politics (for example, Egyptian health policies).

Historian Robert N. Proctor argues on the nature of ignorance as a strategic ploy: "The idea is one that easily lends itself to paranoia: namely, that certain people don't want you to know certain things, or will actively work to organize doubt or uncertainty or misinformation to help maintain (your ignorance)" (Proctor 2008:8). As will be made evident throughout this chapter, and the coming chapters as well, not succumbing to certainty but maintaining uncertainty was often perceived as the safest way to move forward among many of the people that I worked with in Cairo, for example, in relation to medical care. Invoking uncertainty was, in other words, not only reserved for those in power, but also for cartoonists and others.

This chapter sets off empirically at a medical consultation in an outpatient clinic for diabetics in Cairo. Thematically, the chapter begins by looking into the topic of laughter and humor. I have chosen this beginning for the book because it was partly the frequency of laughter during medical consultations in Cairo that pointed me to the most central theme of the book; uncertainty and how it is related to etiologies of type-2 diabetes. Much sociological and anthropological literature on laughter and humor has focused on its dual ability to regenerate structures of power and subordination, as well as to rebel against such structures. Both laughter and humor, in other words, seem to manifest fundamental tensions between liberation and repression, those who laugh and those who are laughed at, the comic and the tragic, release and anxiety (see, for example, Bergson 1911; Carty and Musharbash 2008; Goldstein 2003; Weems 2014).

Sociologist Anton C. Zijderveld captures these tensions in this way: "The shipwrecked person on his lonely island may be the target of many jokes, but he himself has very little reason to laugh" (Zijderveld 1983:3). The ambiguity of laughter and humor is evident also in the very physiological movement of laughter, which greatly resembles that of fear and anxiety (see, for example, Redmond 2008). In this chapter, I make this ambiguity of laughter and humor a focal point, focusing less on the potential power dynamics of the two, and more on the ambiguity of humor and laughter and the uncertainty they both potentially generate. I argue that attempts by authorities and doctors to invoke certainty, for example, in political events and medical facts, were contested through the use of humor and laughter among people in Cairo. Humor and laughter, in other words, provided people with a common space of communication without succumbing to the certainty of specific narratives or so-called facts. I thus argue that humor and laughter were drawn upon by people in Cairo as a way to protect themselves from potential harm. However, it also left them in a state of great uncertainty as to how to move forward in many spheres of everyday life, including in relation to medical advice.

In the first part of the chapter, I examine conversations and laughter in two diabetes consultations in Cairo, focusing specifically on the questioning of medical advice. I draw here on semiotic theories of humor, particularly on the notion of "reversals" (see, for example, Keisalo 2016; Zijderveld 1983). I argue that the semiotic nature of the conversations in these medical consultations often came to resemble something which, essentially, they were not: a laughing matter. In the second part of the chapter, I outline how the tendency to question authorities, so-called facts, and knowledge was not unique to diabetes consultations, but rather a general tendency evident in many spheres of everyday life in Cairo. This came to be seen, for example, in the frequent sharing of conspiracy theories among friends and family, as well as in satirical cartoons published daily in the local newspapers.

In summary, this chapter sets the stage for the following chapters of the book by outlining ways in which uncertainty historically has been drawn upon as a political tool in Egypt to maintain a firm grip on its population – while also illustrating the ways in which uncertainty was invoked by the people I worked with in Cairo as a way to resist this grip in the first place. The arguments of the chapter feed into the overall argument of the book; that whereas such uncertainty was invoked as a way to protect, for example, one's health, it was also perceived to cause experiences of *ḍaghṭ* and thus potentially the onset of type-2 diabetes.

The Diabetes Clinic in Giza (September 2015)

"Why are you here if you don't have diabetes?" Yasmine, a young doctor, asks an older woman sitting across from us. I am sitting next to Yasmine behind the desk in one of the consultation rooms in the clinic. The woman is sitting in one of the lounge chairs opposite the desk. I think she is somewhere in her 60s. She is breathing heavily with her hands on her knees, trying to catch her breath. She closes her eyes for a few seconds and then wipes away drops of sweat from her forehead.

Yasmine looks intensely at the woman. Waiting. Still out of breath, the woman finally asks Yasmine if she can measure her blood pressure.

Yasmine sighs. "This is a diabetes clinic," she says. "For people with diabetes." The woman doesn't respond.

"There is a pharmacy down the street," Yasmine says, and explains that the woman can get her blood pressure measured there. The woman ignores Yasmine's advice.

"I am traveling," the woman then says. Yasmine looks at her with a rather blank stare. The woman explains that she often has her blood pressure and blood sugar levels measured.

"Not here though," Yasmine responds.

The woman continues, "I recently had a blood sugar level of 108. Is that normal?"

Yasmine says, "It's fine."

The woman changes topics. "I just had eye surgery," she says. Now, I can see clearly." She stretches out her hands and fingers in front of her as if she could not see them clearly before.

Yasmine has turned to examine the computer screen next to her, scrolling down the list of patients waiting outside. The woman is still talking about her recent eye surgery. She asks Yasmine if she has seen a specific commercial on TV for a particular doctor. "He did my surgery. He has a clinic in Masr Gadida.[1] Do you know the place?" the woman asks.

Yasmine shuffles some papers around the desk and mutters that she has indeed heard of the place.

"It's a famous hospital," the woman adds.

Yasmine nods and smiles briefly. The woman thanks Yasmine for listening, "*Allāh khalīkī, Allāh khalīkī*, May God protect you." The woman slowly tries to get up from the chair, but immediately falls back into it. She still sounds out of breath.

"It's nice to rest under the air-conditioner," she then says.

Yasmine politely tells the woman to stay for as long as she needs to. The woman silently stares at her own folded hands for a while before repeating her recent fasting blood sugar measurement of 108 mg/dL.

"Are you sure it's fine?" she asks Yasmine.

Yasmine reassures the woman with a mix of English and Arabic, "*Da* safe."

The woman finally gets up from her chair. "*Da* safe," the woman repeats while slowly walking out of the consultation room.

As soon as the woman is out of the door, Yasmine turns to me, and bursts out laughing. "She was so sweet, but she didn't even have diabetes!" she says to me in English.

A man in his 50s enters the consultation room, interrupting Yasmine's laughter. His movements are swift. He gives us a big smile, revealing a mouth with barely any teeth. He hands Yasmine a piece of paper from the lab, and Yasmine quickly asks the man for his medical history and current treatment. He explains that he has been dealing with type-2 diabetes for the past ten years and that he takes insulin in the morning. He fishes out an ampule of insulin from his pocket, and shows it to Yasmine.

"And?" Yasmine looks at the man upon examining the ampule.

"*Bas*, that's it," he says.

"You cannot possibly take this type of insulin only once a day. It only works for 12 hours, you have to take it twice a day," Yasmine says. Yasmine turns to look at the man's lab results. His measurements are very high, indicating that he is not taking enough insulin.

The man starts explaining that his sister has diabetes, but that she only takes insulin once a day. "That's better," he says.

Yasmine starts explaining that not all insulin is the same; there are many types of insulin. "You have to take your type of insulin twice a day," she says.

"But I only eat once a day, breakfast," the man says.

"You only eat breakfast, and then nothing until the next morning?" Yasmine asks, clearly skeptical.

"Correct," the man responds.

Yasmine shakes her head and tells the man that he should eat something at least twice a day. And take his insulin twice a day. The man doesn't respond. Yasmine sighs. She looks at the computer. She then asks the man if he has any problems with his eyes.

"No," he says. Yasmine checks a box on the computer stating that the man does in fact have problems with his eyes. She then gives him a referral to an eye doctor down the hall.

Yasmine moves on to the next question on the screen. "Do you eat more or less than usual?"

"I eat A LOT," the man says. Yasmine looks sharply at the man, and the two of them burst out laughing.

"How do you eat a lot when you only have breakfast?" Yasmine asks, before throwing herself back into her chair. The man responds with a mere chuckle.

Yasmine finally asks the man if he is taking any other medicine.

"Yes, B-vitamins," he responds.

"By pill or needle?" Yasmine asks.

"No, pills!" the man responds quickly. Yasmine looks at him and says that taking the vitamins is better by needle.

"I don't like needles," he says.

"But you take insulin?" Yasmine responds.

The man starts explaining that he goes to the pharmacy every morning to get his injection of insulin because he is afraid to do it himself. The walk there is tiring, "*ḍaghṭ kathīr*, it's a lot of pressure," he says. He mutters something.

Yasmine sighs, "So this is why you only take your insulin once a day?"

"No," he says.

Yasmine sharply responds, "You are tired because your blood sugar is so high from eating a lot and from a lack of insulin."

The man quietly responds, "No, I am tired from walking to the pharmacy."

The two go on for a while. Once the man is out of the door, Yasmine turns to me and rolls her eyes. She says, "That man is going to kill himself!" She then bursts out laughing once again while shaking her head in what seems to be disbelief.

A Laughing Matter

The above consultations took place in an outpatient clinic for diabetics at a public hospital in the working-class neighborhood of Giza (situated in the southwestern part of Cairo). The multinational medical company Novo Nordisk (Novo) had recently renovated the clinic, and it was thus bright and shiny, furnished with state-of-the-art medical equipment, in stark contrast to the rest of the hospital (I will return to unfold the engagements of Novo with this clinic in Chapter 6).

The consultations illustrate the course of most of the diabetes consultations that I attended during my fieldwork in Cairo. Most were constituted to some degree by what can be described as parallel-running tracks of meanings and perspectives, resulting in conversations, questions, and answers that, at times, seemed to consist mostly of contradictions and inconsistencies. Take some examples from above. Comment: "This is a diabetes clinic." Response: "I am traveling." Statement #1: "I only eat breakfast." Statement #2: "I eat a lot." Question: "Do you have problems with your eyes?" Answer: "No." Response: "Problems with sight" ticked off as a symptom in the patient's file, patient receives a referral to an eye doctor.

Most of the medical consultations that I attended in Cairo were constituted by similar elements of contradictions and inconsistencies, at times manifested in downright disagreements over etiologies and treatments. Despite such disagreements, most of the people that I worked with in Cairo who were diagnosed with type-2 diabetes kept consulting a doctor on a regular basis. Returning to the above account, in Yasmine's perspective, the man in particular seemed reluctant to accept the doctoral advice given to him; to eat twice a day and to take his insulin twice a day. The woman, on the other hand, was seeking medical advice, and re-advice, it seemed, but was not actually sick with diabetes. So why had she come to the clinic in the first place?

Throughout my fieldwork in Cairo, I heard countless stories of corrupt and poor treatment in all spheres of the Egyptian healthcare system, both first-hand accounts as well as stories from various media outlets. Stories included issues in relation to medicine, such as the very handling of pharmaceuticals, treatment with expired products, and cases in which some medicine did not contain the actual ingredients that they were being sold as (I will elaborate on this particular topic of medical drugs in Chapter 4).

Many patients and members of the families that I worked with the most, as well as healthcare personnel, further told stories of people contracting infections and other health problems from the poor hygiene in hospitals and clinics, including the use of unsterile and broken equipment during examinations and surgeries. In Maha's family (whom I will introduce more thoroughly in the coming chapter), four of her paternal aunts and uncles, for example, had been diagnosed with hepatitis C. All of them connected their point of contraction with surgeries performed at various public hospitals in Cairo.

The bad hygiene and the poor physical conditions of public hospitals were often topics of conversation in the families that I worked with in Cairo. These were also mirrored in the stories of others published in various local and social media outlets. During my first phase of fieldwork in Cairo in 2015, a Facebook group run by a group of Egyptian doctors surfaced, posting pictures of poor conditions in public hospitals across Egypt. The pictures included images of cats and snakes camping out in hospital beds, dried-out blood and feces on floors and walls, and doctors performing surgery in the dark, using manual respiration devices and assisted only by the light from cell phones. This resembled my own observations in the various hospitals and clinics that I frequented in Cairo; power cuts and the lack of functional generators, for example, were frequent in these facilities as well.

In addition to the poor hygiene and physical conditions of public hospitals, many of the doctors and patients that I encountered told stories of a very corrupt healthcare system in which bribing healthcare personnel in order to receive proper treatment was common. Furthermore, medical misconduct was widespread. I heard many cases, for example, of patients being treated for ailments that they did not actually have, but that required expensive testing and treatment, from which doctors and others profited greatly. I knew several women who had been told that their pregnancies were ectopic pregnancies, requiring immediate surgery, yet, when consulting different doctors, it turned out that this was not the case at all. Similarly, I spoke to a man who supposedly had a kidney removed at a young age, only to discover later in life that he still had both his kidneys (despite a surgical scar and a medical bill to prove the contrary) (see also Hamdy 2012 and Inhorn 1994 for similar accounts of medical misconduct in Egypt).

The poor and corrupt condition of the Egyptian healthcare system was often depicted in satirical cartoons published in various local newspapers. One such cartoon by cartoonist Abdullah, for example, addressed a supposed outbreak of an unknown virus (and the death of three children). The cartoon was published in the privately owned newspaper *Al-Masry Al-Youm* on March 20, 2017. The cartoon depicts a hepatitis C virus telling another "mysterious" virus," "Mysterious or not, I guarantee you will have a good time in this country." Whereas the cartoon spoke to a specific outbreak, on a more general note, it addressed the poor state of the Egyptian healthcare system which enabled the wide spread of viruses such as hepatitis C or this current "mysterious" virus. Adding a twist to this story, the Egyptian Ministry of Health, in fact, claimed that the "mysterious virus" had never existed, but that rumors of the virus had been spread by Muslim Brotherhood websites (opponents of the regime).

Anthropologist Marcia Inhorn has traced the current healthcare system in Egypt back to European colonialism and military expansion in the country, arguing that the British occupation in Egypt in the late 19th century reversed many reforms of the time. Admission to medical school came to be based, for example, on upper-class status and the ability to pay tuition. Medical practice was turned into a trade-for-profit, and medical education, and in many instances the communication with patients, was no longer conducted in Arabic, but in English (Inhorn 1994:64–5). From her work in Egypt in the 1990s, Inhorn argues, "The deleterious ramifications of British imperial rule are still remarkably evident in Egyptian biomedicine today" (Inhorn 1994:65). Political scientist Timothy Mitchell has since argued on a more general note that the presence of foreign powers has continued in Egypt past the time of colonialism by way of international organizations such as the International Monetary Fund, the World Bank, and USAID. Mitchell argues that these institutions have exercised great influence over Egyptian politics, economy, and society, including the organization of the healthcare sector and medical training (Mitchell 2002:211).

As will be made evident throughout this book, Egyptian medical practice can be characterized largely as a trade-for-profit in the sense that large sums of money are paid to access doctors and treatments, retrieve and hold hospital beds and, for example, undergo certain examinations – whether by way of bribes in the supposedly free-of-charge public healthcare system, or by way of paying to access expensive private care facilities. A grave example of this appeared in Mohamed's family (whom the reader will be introduced to below) in the spring of 2017, as his uncle suddenly fell ill from an unknown condition. After hours in the emergency room at one of the public university hospitals in Cairo, he passed away. The doctors in the emergency room had refused to admit him to the intensive care unit in the hospital upon realizing that the family could not mobilize an unofficial payment to a senior doctor in the ward. I later learned from Taher, a young doctor who will be introduced further in Chapter 4, that this was common practice across public hospitals in Cairo. Taher recounted several examples similar to the one of Mohamed's uncle of patients dying prematurely in the emergency room because senior doctors would not admit them to the intensive care unit – despite available beds and equipment. "They are keeping the bed for someone more important, someone with stars on their shoulders, someone who can pay with money and connections," he explained.

Gaps in social class are often evident among patients and doctors in the public healthcare system, as most doctors belong to the wealthier segments of Egyptian society – whereas most of the patients frequenting the public healthcare system do not. Doctors do not simply belong to the wealthier segments because of their status as doctors, but because most of them stem from upper or upper-middle class families in the first place. These are families that have the financial means to send their children to private school, as well as to assist them in other ways to get high scores in their final exams. Such high scores (as well as a combination of hard work and, sometimes, I hear, nepotism) allow these children to access medical school at one of the free public universities in Egypt, or to enter medical school at one of the expensive private universities.

In summary, the Egyptian public healthcare system that I encountered during my fieldwork in Cairo was characterized greatly by medical misconduct, corruption, and class division, both with regard to patients' access to healthcare and in regard to the general relations between patients and doctors.

Past stories of consulting doctors and seeking treatment in the Egyptian public healthcare system, as well as widespread and contradicting stories in the media, had been so confusing and discouraging to many of the people that I knew in Cairo that "doubt about the transparency of motives" seemed more than "reasonable," to cite Asad, whose overall arguments I presented in the introduction to this chapter (Asad 2012:275). As a result, my field notes are full of people, some that I knew well and some that I merely met in passing, who questioned and debated medical advice given by doctors with their relatives, friends, colleagues, and others: What is this doctor's agenda?

I might also mention here that hospital employees in Egypt have occasionally been accused of nullifying or falsifying evidence of state violence and police brutality by refusing to document bruises and other such evidence in official files and death certificates. Some hospital employees have even been accused of purposely mistreating demonstrators during the Arab Spring of 2011 (see also Hamdy and Bayoumi 2016). Such stories further added to the reluctance to merely trust in doctors among the people that I worked with in Cairo, though others recounted stories also of heroic healthcare personnel who put themselves in danger to treat wounded demonstrators during the uprisings in 2011 and later in 2013.

Returning once again to the above consultations, I did not have the opportunity to discuss the consultations with the two patients involved. Based on many similar consultations, I do suspect that the woman came to the clinic to retrieve a second opinion on a blood sugar measurement that she had most likely paid for elsewhere, not trusting that the measurement was within the normal range. It is also possible that she came to retrieve reassurance that she had chosen a good hospital for her eye surgery, though she ended up mostly reassuring herself ("Now I can see clearly"). It is also possible that she came to the clinic simply to enjoy a moment of cool air, peace, and quiet. This was not uncommon at this clinic, as the state-of-the-art facility (including the air-conditioners) stood in stark contrast to the surrounding neighborhood and climate. Most likely, the woman came to the clinic for a combination of all of these things.

Anthropologist Sherine Hamdy argues from her research among kidney patients in Egypt, "In Egypt the major issues in biomedical debates are not about the legitimacy of biomedicine itself but rather about the ethics of its application" (Hamdy 2012:36). This sums up the sentiment that I picked up among the people that I was working with in Cairo as well; few people seemed to question the legitimacy of biomedicine as such, though most questioned the ethics and motives of the doctors, nurses, pharmacists, pharmaceutical companies, authorities, and others involved in the business surrounding the realm of biomedicine. This perhaps explains why the man described above chose to consult Yasmine and the clinic, despite his reluctance to follow her advice.

In other words, the man did not seem to question biomedicine and the potential positive effects of medicine as such (after all he did go to the clinic and he did supposedly take both insulin and B-vitamins). Rather, the man seemed to question the advice given to him by Yasmine to take his insulin twice a day (his skepticism, most likely, being caused by the contradicting advice that he had received from his aunt and from his own personal experiences of the effects on his health of having to walk to the pharmacist to get his daily injections of insulin). In fact, several of the people that I worked with in Cairo who were diagnosed with type-2 diabetes ended up taking different medicines or dosages of medicine than had been advised by their doctors. This was possible because most medicine can be bought in Egypt without a prescription (I will address all of these issues more thoroughly in Chapter 6).

Questions and disagreements between patients and healthcare personnel did result in many cases of verbal (and even physical) fights and tears, but as evident in the above consultations (and many more throughout my field notes), they also resulted in a lot of laughter. Patients and relatives thus laughed at each other and at the doctor; doctors and patients laughed with and at each other; doctors and relatives laughed at the patients; patients and relatives laughed after the consultations (at the doctor and at themselves); and doctors laughed when patients had left the office. So why was this all such a laughing matter?

Several social scientists have written about humor in an Egyptian context. In the 1980s, for example, political scientist Samer S. Shehata argued that humor in Egypt was put to use as a relief from political oppression and that political jokes could be examined as a window into public opinion (Shehata 1992); social scientists Mohamed M. Helmy and Sabine Frerichs argued upon the uprisings in 2011 that humor in Egypt turned out not only to provide relief and a window into public opinion, but also to provide the grounds for an actual revolution (Helmy and Frerichs 2013); anthropologists Mari Norbakk (Norbakk 2018) and Farha Ghannam (Ghannam 2013) have separately focused within recent years on the ways in which humor is put to use as a form of social capital especially among men in Egypt; and, finally, anthropologist Chihab El Khachab has worked to emphasize the ambiguous nature of humor in Egypt – challenging the notion that humor reflects an authentic voice as such, emphasizing instead the ways in which humor is read differently depending on individuals, contexts and points in time (Khachab 2017).

Along the lines of El Khachab, much of the general social literature on humor attempts to understand the semiotics of humor; essentially what makes us laugh. This literature focuses especially on the semiotic notion of "reversals," a playing with meanings by a constant shift of perspectives (see, for example, Weems 2014 for an overview of some of this literature). Anthropologist Marianna Keisalo, for example, argues that comedic figures "play with, combine, or shift between opposite traits, actions and perspectives" (Keisalo 2016:62). "It seems that all humor has an aspect of incongruity, such as bringing together elements that do not 'go together,' or involving a double framing that makes the message ambiguous" (Keisalo 2018:118–19). Similarly, sociologist William B. Cameron once argued that, "Many jokes derive their effect by contrasting two different frames of reference in which something which would be appropriate to one is mistaken and inappropriate to the other" (Cameron 1963:85).

Returning to the above consultations at the diabetes clinic in Giza, this was somewhat the sentiment that I was initially left with. I did not perceive the laughter during these or other consultations to be merely a matter of resistance (see, for example, Douglas 1966; Goldstein 2003; Scott 1985 for elaborations of the relation between laughter and resistance), nor simply a matter of resignation. Rather, I argue, the laughter appeared also to be a matter of reversals. The consistent clash of shifting and opposing perspectives, in other words, resulted in conversations of seeming absurdities and contradictions, resembling something they were essentially not: a joke. The conversations evolved in such ways, I argue, because doctors were not merely accepted as experts or authorities to be trusted. Medical knowledge and so-called facts were questioned by patients and their relatives; uncertainty maintained.

Keisalo quotes famous American stand-up comedian Louis C. K., for framing a good joke as an "epistemological problem" in which one gets "trapped" (Keisalo 2016:73). Perhaps this was why medical consultations such as the ones described above had the potential to suddenly transform into a laughing matter – patients and doctors found themselves trapped in an epistemological problem, laughter an appropriate response to this "problem." In other words, laughter during medical consultations such as those depicted above can be viewed, I argue, as a response to the uncertainty evident in the semiotic reversals during those consultations.

A Café in Dokki (June 2015)

We are sitting at a sidewalk café in Dokki. It's nighttime and Mohamed's friend, Mina, is with us. Music is drifting from the speakers. It's the Egyptian Frank Sinatra, according to Mohamed. I don't catch the singer's actual name. We are talking about the last few years, especially the uprisings in 2011 and their aftermath during Morsi's presidency. Mohamed turns to us, laughing, preparing to tell us a story.

"You know, at the time of the big sit-ins in Giza and Rabaa I had an American friend, Jason, who was totally oblivious to what was happening outside his hotel, so he decided to go for a walk around Giza. He was like walking around with his backpack and camera, just strolling the streets."

Mina and I laugh as Mohamed mimics how Jason was walking around with his backpack like a schoolbag, holding on to the straps like a child. Mohamed continues the story.

"A group of men thought Jason looked really suspicious and accused him of being a spy. Jason got really scared and tried convincing them that he was Russian, not American, because he thought it was better being a Russian. However, they found his American passport while rummaging through his backpack, so they detained him, forced him into their car, and finally took him to the police station."

I look at Mohamed rather shocked, empathizing with this unknown Jason. Mohamed continues the story.

"I was at home sleeping when my phone rang, and this serious voice asks me if I am Mohamed Mustafa. My first thought was 'what did I do?'" Mohamed jokingly makes a scared face. "But then I heard Jason in the background trying to communicate with the police officer. He handed Jason the phone and Jason was almost crying when he told me they were holding him at the police station." Mohamed looks more serious now.

I am listening intensely to the story, while Mina is sipping his Pepsi, looking much less impressed. Mohamed continues the story, now on a lighter note.

"So, I went to the police station as fast as I could. They had put Jason in an interrogation room and given him a cup of Nescafé to try to calm him down. Not Arabic coffee, but *Nescafé* ... because he is a foreigner, to try and make him feel more like home!" Mohamed bursts out laughing. "The police officer told me they weren't going to let him out before I got there, because chances were some other men would detain him. So, I took him home, and he left Egypt like a few days later."

"Wow, that's a really good story," Mina says.

"Yeah for Mohamed, not so much for Jason," I add.

They both laugh and nod in agreement.

Mohamed orders another round of Pepsis. Mina then asks Mohamed, "Hey, do you remember when we were teenagers and this theory was going around that Pepsi is actually an abbreviation for 'Pays Every Penny To Israel' or something?" We all laugh.

Mohamed adds, "Yeah, and Coca Cola in Arabic spelled backwards reads '*La Mohamed, La Mekka*, no to Mohammed, no to Mecca.'" We laugh again.

"That one is actually true," Mohamed says. After a while he adds, "Egypt is the land of conspiracy theories." I nod.

"Did you hear the theory about the earthquake yesterday? And the sandstorm?" Mohamed turns to me. I shake my head no. "People are saying that what happened is really God's anger, because so many Egyptians changed their Facebook profile picture to rainbow colors now that same-sex marriage is allowed in the States."

I shake my head no again, "No, I didn't hear this."

Mohamed nods. "Yeah, really. People are saying this."

I change the topic and ask about the recent assassination of a public prosecutor. (His car was blown up somewhere in Heliopolis and he died immediately.) I tell Mohamed and Mina that I heard someone from the Muslim Brotherhood did it. Mohamed says, "Yeah, no ... probably Sisi is behind it, but they *want* you to believe that it is the Muslim Brotherhood."

I nod, "Yeah, okay." We order more Pepsis and chat about other topics before Mohamed turns to me and asks, "Do you remember the whole thing with the cartoons?"

I nod and say, "Yes, of course." Cartoons of the Prophet were published in a Danish newspaper in 2005, causing a major diplomatic crisis between Muslim communities across the globe and Denmark.

"I went demonstrating in front of the Danish Embassy!" Mohamed says.

Mina looks up, "Ha! Me too!"

I smile and tell them good for them. I picture the two of them in their late teens, standing in front of the Danish Embassy in the upscale neighborhood of Zamalek. I then ask how they managed to demonstrate in front of the embassy which is in an apartment building on a rather narrow street. They both laugh and Mina says, "Yeah, it was quite crowded."

I tell them that I heard a theory that former President Mubarak orchestrated the turmoil surrounding the cartoons of the Prophet in Egypt, in order to draw attention away from himself and the upcoming presidential elections in Egypt at the time (the first presidential elections ever in Egypt).

Mohamed looks at me with a blank stare as if scattered pieces are finally falling into place. "Wow," he says. "You are right ..." He ponders for a bit before he dramatically exclaims, "I feel so fooled!"

We all laugh, and quickly move on to another round of Pepsis and stories.

Conspiracy Theorizing

I knew Mohamed initially from his mother, whom I was introduced to at the beginning of my fieldwork in 2015. Mohamed's mother was diagnosed with type-2 diabetes, and had been for some years.

Mina was Mohamed's close friend, and the three of us met on several occasions, chatting about this and that, including current affairs in Egypt. Mohamed and Mina were both in their late 20s, and worked as translators and fixers for various international media outlets. "Egypt is the land of conspiracy theories," Mohamed expressed in the above conversation after we had touched, firstly, on a story of strangers deeming an unknown Jason to be a conspiring character, and, secondly, on American soda companies seemingly conspiring against Muslim and Arab communities around the globe.

Throughout the above night we moved on to other stories involving named politicians, officials, activists, weather phenomena, and even God, continuously raising questions of what had *actually* happened during the recent sandstorm and earthquake, or what was the *actual* underlying cause of the assassination of the public prosecutor. "Did you hear ...?" "Do you remember ...?" "... or something?" Hence, the questioning of authorities and stories, the reversing of truths, were not unique to diabetes consultations, but a tendency that I observed in many spheres throughout my fieldwork in Cairo. Picking up the above story where I left it, I forgot where I had heard the theory that former President Mubarak orchestrated the turmoil in Egypt surrounding the cartoons of the Prophet. My guess is that I first heard it in the Danish media at the time of the turmoil. I recounted the theory to Mohamed and Mina mainly to tease the two, not having done any research on the matter myself (and thus with no real ability to evaluate whether I found the theory feasible at all). Nonetheless, it worked: Mohamed felt "fooled."

Looking back, Mohamed's comment, and our subsequent laughter, depicted much of the unresolved nature of conversations such as the one above, as well as those that I had observed during the diabetes consultations. Did Mohamed laugh, for example, because he had truly felt "fooled," and essentially embarrassed that he had not sufficiently questioned the motives of President Mubarak, or did he, perhaps, rather laugh at me, the Dane, clearly trying to wash her hands of any responsibility in relation to the turmoil? Was Mohamed's laughter sarcastic? A snort, a snicker? Or was it perhaps a nervous giggle? I am not sure. Either way, the laughter of Mohamed, Mina, and myself roared in many different directions throughout the night.

Take the initial story of Jason, the American. Mohamed sets the scene well, painting an image of Jason as a rather naïve, trusting young man, who clearly grew up in a different world than the one he wandered into in Giza. Jason contrasts the crowd of Egyptian men, who, full of mistrust and suspicion, rummage through Jason's backpack, detain him, and end up taking him to the police station on accusations that he is an American spy. Examining the above account, both Mohamed, Mina, and I laughed at Mohamed's initial description of Jason. Yet, as the story evolves, and our empathy shifts to Jason, our laughter dies out, perhaps, in a brief moment of disbelief and anticipation. Our laughter picks up again as Mohamed enters the story, emphasizing an act of care and consideration carried out by an otherwise brutally depicted police force (serving Jason Nescafé rather than Arabic coffee, trying to "make him feel more like home"). Zijderveld argues on the nature of humor, "Ambiguity is the essence of humour. Therefore, the tragic and the comic are often hard to distinguish." He elaborates, "The clash of frames of meaning is, as it were, a little drama which unfolds before our eyes, and leads to a cathartic smile or relieving laugh" (Zijderveld 1983:23).

I believe that Mohamed's story mostly served to ridicule the foolishness of the Egyptian crowd who had at first scared Jason, then detained him, and, finally, forced Mohamed out of bed and all the way to the police station in Giza. I emphasize the story here, because much of the laughter throughout the above conversation was not merely aimed at authorities, police, politicians, and the like. Rather, it was aimed also at those who actually believed in certain conspiracy theories, including the crowds in Giza or the teenage selves of Mohamed and Mina (who in their younger years, for example, had been preoccupied with an allegedly bittersweet relation between Pepsi and Israel). Yet, the ambiguity remained of what Mohamed and Mina actually believed themselves, when they were laughing at the theory of Pepsi and Israel, but maintaining the story of Coca Cola ("This one is actually true"). The laughter released upon the questioning of stories and theories cemented the unresolved nature of these theories, which were rarely deemed "actually true." The laughter neither confirmed nor dismissed the theories, but rather left a roaring question mark throughout the conversation.

The ambiguity of humor and laughter, I argue, is why it was so often put to use among the people I worked with in Cairo, for example, in satirical cartoons, at cafés in Dokki as well as during medical consultations in the public healthcare system. Humor and laughter were both spontaneous reactions to uncertainty – semiotic reversals and contradictions – but also invoked to generate and maintain uncertainty, for example, as to one's political beliefs and understandings: Whom are we laughing at and why?

Recounting different stories than those told by the Egyptian authorities can be quite a dangerous business in Egypt. I have both read reports and heard first-hand accounts of journalists, researchers, lawyers, and others who have been arrested (or who have disappeared), allegedly for challenging official stories released by the Egyptian authorities. Throughout my fieldwork stays in Egypt, the Egyptian authorities regularly accused both individuals and entire news outlets of "spreading lies" and "supporting terrorism" (Michaelson 2017). In the summer of 2017, more than 20 news websites were as a result blocked by the authorities in an attempt to prevent access from within Egypt. These websites included Al-Jazeera and the Arabic version of the Huffington Post, as well as Egyptian Mada Masr. However, as evident throughout this chapter, such actions by authorities did not simply silence people, but did make them communicate, for example, through the ambiguity of humor and laughter.

Anthropologists Maria Frederika Malmström (Malmström 2019) and Talal Asad (Asad 2012), as well as political scientist Mona El-Ghobashy (El-Ghobashy 2021), have separately written about the ways in which uncertainty historically, as well as during the past decade in Egypt, has been drawn upon by the Egyptian state apparatus as a way to control the Egyptian population. This has manifested, for example, in an omnipresent sentiment among many Egyptians – evident also throughout my research – of being surveilled by the Egyptian intelligence service, *il-mukhābarāt*, and never feeling quite sure as to whether or not one's behavior can be viewed as problematic or downright criminal.

Anthropologist Linda Green has previously captured such sentiments from her own experiences with fear and surveillance in early 1990s Guatemala, "The plight of Joseph K in Franz Kafka's *Trial* flashed through my mind, the character accused of a crime for which he must defend himself but about which he could get no information. 'I didn't do anything wrong; I must not look guilty,' I told myself over and over" (Green 1994:244–5). As should be evident throughout the above, humor and laughter provided the people I worked with in Cairo with a common space for communication about issues that were contested without succumbing to the certainty of specific narratives or beliefs; whereas uncertainty was generated by the Egyptian state to maintain a firm grip on its population, these same methods were drawn upon by the people I came across in Cairo to resist this grip in the first place. This mechanism has been exemplified throughout the above and was exemplified also in another satirical drawing by cartoonist Anwar published on the last day of the 2018 presidential elections in Egypt in the privately owned newspaper *Al-Masry Al-Youm*. The cartoon depicts two doctors and a patient in a psychiatric hospital, one doctor telling the other doctor, "We caught him saying that he doesn't know who will win the election ..." Once again, the ambiguity of the narrative of the cartoon makes it a space of communication about issues contested in the public sphere. The cartoon may be read either as a comment on the uncertainties that a fair presidential election may generate within a population, the patient sick with concerns about the future. On the other hand, the cartoon may also express the sentiment that the outcome of the elections was predetermined (in favor of President al-Sisi), overall depicting the paradox that one ought not to question the position of President al-Sisi (it could be dangerous), yet, this is exactly what is done both by the patient in the cartoon and by the cartoonist himself.

As mentioned at the beginning of this chapter, the physical movement of laughter greatly resembles that of anxiety, for example, in increased inhalation and expiration, a sense of suffocation, dilating of the pupils and blood flowing to the face (see, for example, Redmond 2008). In other words, laughter as a physical movement embodies the ambiguity intrinsic to the semiotics of humor, the simultaneous presence of the tragic and the comic, "Why laughter is so close to tears," in the words of anthropologist Michael Jackson (Jackson 2002:170). Throughout the above, I have argued that the semiotics of humor, and the subsequent physical response of laughter, were not merely present throughout my fieldwork in Cairo in situations that were meant to be funny (such as in satirical cartoons, and, partly, in conversations revolving around conspiracy theories). They were also present during medical consultations. Maintaining uncertainty, for example, in relation to medical advice or political beliefs provided some form of relief, but it simultaneously generated further tension as questions were left unanswered, facts were never fully determined, medical etiologies and treatments never felt quite certain. In similar ways, I argue, humor and laughter simultaneously provided relief and tension.

At one point during my fieldwork in Cairo I asked Maha, whom you will be introduced to in the following chapter, why there was such an overwhelming number of Egyptian comedies being produced by the Egyptian movie industry and so few social and political dramas; surely there were issues to be addressed? "We laugh and then we cry," she responded in relation to the comedies, pointing to the ambiguous nature of these movies – relief and tension. "Laughter does not just arise from fear, but can also lead to it," anthropologists John Carty and Yasmine Musharbash fittingly argue (Carty and Musharbash 2008:214).

Anthropologist Katherine Ewing has outlined how people tend to present multiple, conflicting narratives, yet continue to live under an illusion of wholeness. People function, she argues, in conflicting semiotic environments because uncertainties and inconsistencies are transformed into overall experiences of coherence and wholeness (Ewing 1990). Anthropologist Samuli Schielke draws on these perspectives by Ewing when unfolding how young men in Egypt present shifting, and at times contradicting, sets of views. However, Schielke argues, they are not living under an illusion of wholeness, but rather they are left very aware of these shifts and contradictions (Schielke 2009). Evident throughout the above, I observed the same kind of awareness among the people that I was working with in Cairo, as well as a tendency to actively engage with such contrasting points of views as a way to get by in everyday life.

Pierce once argued, "Doubt is an uneasy and dissatisfied state from which we struggle to free ourselves and pass into the state of belief" (Pierce 1998:125). Along similar lines, Pelkmans more recently argued that doubt brings forth a sort of "restlessness" (Pelkmans 2016:499), having previously argued that doubt possesses an immediate need to be "tamed, sidelined or transformed" (Pelkmans 2013:20). Returning to the ethnographic accounts presented in this chapter, the very opposite seemed to be true for Mohamed and Mina, as well as the patients visiting Yasmine. "Belief" rather than "doubt" appeared to constitute the "uneasy" or "restless" state of being for them all. Thus, Mohamed, Mina, and others struggled to free themselves, not of their doubts, but rather of attempts by the Egyptian authorities, doctors, and others to uphold certain and definite beliefs ("They *want* you to believe that it is the Muslim Brotherhood," Mohamed questioned my understanding of what had happened to the public prosecutor).

In summary, rather than accepting truths as presented, for example, by doctors and other healthcare personnel, patients consistently questioned medical explanations and treatments. This is evident in the two diabetes consultations presented in this chapter, and it will be made more evident in the following chapters of this book as well.

"Enough! *Khalāṣ!*" Ahmed Laughs (August 2015)

"Do you want to see something?" Ahmed asks. A smile spreads across his face.

I smile and nod, "Always."

We are sitting together in the garden of a villa in Maadi, an upscale neighborhood where Ahmed works as a gardener. He fetches his Nokia phone from the pocket of his worn-out jeans. He wipes off the dust from its screen with the bottom of his t-shirt. He flips through the photos on his phone, and finally shows me a blurry picture of himself and another young gardener from down the street, Mahmoud. They are swimming in a pool. I ask Ahmed if they went on holiday.

Ahmed laughs, "No, one of the families down the street went away on a holiday. Mahmoud and I went swimming in their pool one night when they were gone. *Don't tell anyone*," he whispers.

I laugh as we flip through the other pictures of their secret night swim. I know that Ahmed lives close by in Dar al Salam; close to this upscale neighborhood of Maadi in kilometers, but a world apart in terms of resources and social class.

"It was my first time in a swimming pool," Ahmed adds.

Ahmed puts away his phone, and asks me about my research. He hands me a cup of tea, as I tell him about the clinic in Giza. I ask Ahmed about diabetes as well.

"A person with diabetes has too much sugar in the blood," Ahmed says. I nod at the familiar explanation while sipping the sugary mint tea. I ask Ahmed how people end up with "too much" sugar in their blood.

"Life in Egypt, especially in Cairo, it's really difficult, there is so much pressure here, *ḍaghṭ kathīr*," he says. He adds, "You know, pressure from life, *ḍaghṭ min il-ḥayā*, will result in pressure in your blood, *ḍaghṭ fī il-dam*, right?"

I keep nodding and sipping my tea, while asking Ahmed more questions about diabetes. I ask "Why? *Leh?*" and "How? *Izzay?*" "What exactly causes pressure in the blood?"

Ahmed starts listing various risk factors. Depression. Feeling sad or worried. Nervous. Aggressive. Angry. Being scared. "For example, if a pregnant woman is very sad or scared, the baby might get diabetes," Ahmed explains. After a short while he adds, "This is why it's important to laugh a lot and not think too much, *matafakkarsh kathīr*. You know Egyptians have these sayings? *Mata'ṣabsh kathīr*. Don't get angry too often. *Matitkhān'ish ma' mirātak kathīr*. Don't fight too much with your wife." Ahmed sips his tea, focusing in on his cup. "This is also why you should drink tea. You can't drink tea when you are angry. You have to relax when you drink tea."

I ask Ahmed if factors such as weight and food intake can cause diabetes. He laughs and says that I got it all wrong. "You can't get diabetes because you are fat!"

We both laugh at my assumption. I then start asking Ahmed about politics.

"Politics in Egypt is really bad. There is a lot of corruption … surely you know this already," he says.

I ask if the corruption is worse today than before the revolution.

Ahmed points at a wooden garden gate in front of us. "Before the revolution, the President would maybe take a piece of wood for himself. There would still be a door. Today, the President will take the whole door. He doesn't care."

We laugh fondly at the comparison, picturing President al-Sisi walking off with the wooden gate. I look at the villa behind us and then ask Ahmed if people in Maadi joined in on the demonstrations during the revolution in 2011.

Ahmed laughs and says, "Nooo," while clicking his tongue. "*They don't benefit from political change*," he whispers.

I lower my voice and ask if he can elaborate a bit further. He lets out a big laugh and throws his hands in the air. "Enough! *Khalāṣ!* You are going to give me diabetes with all these questions!"[2]

Summary

Ahmed, who was in his early 30s, had worked his entire life in the garden as described above, first, as a child along with his father, later, upon his father's passing, on his own. He had recently married, and become the father of a little girl. In addition, he had three sisters, all of whom had married much earlier, and two younger brothers, who were still living at home with their mother. Ahmed was the oldest son, and thus financially responsible, not only for his wife and daughter, but also for his mother and his two brothers. Ahmed often stayed at his mother's house, caring greatly for her health and wellbeing. When Ahmed's father passed away, his mother had fallen ill with type-2 diabetes, "*min il-zaʿil*," from the sadness, they both explained.

Despite all of these responsibilities, Ahmed always seemed happy and lighthearted. Conversations with him were full of laughter and reminders to "not think too much" or to not "get angry too often." Much of this laughter was triggered by a great many semiotic reversals, contradictions, and inconsistencies. Ahmed thus recounts in words and pictures how he and Mahmoud had fooled their rich employers by taking a night-time dip in their swimming pool. He serves me sugary mint tea as he relates the condition of diabetes to someone having "too much sugar in their blood." He dismisses the notion that food intake and obesity are in any way related to diabetes, causing us both to laugh, but for different reasons (Ahmed at me, I at Ahmed). He paints an image of President al-Sisi strolling off with a worthless wooden gate, literally funny, figuratively speaking not so funny. He laughs as I propose that the posh people of Maadi would ever take part in a revolutionary act, and we both laugh as Ahmed elegantly tells me to back off, indicating that I might give him diabetes from the *ḍaghṭ*, pressure, of all of my questions.

In the following chapter, I will unfold how factors such as those outlined by Ahmed in the above were widely known to cause *ḍaghṭ*, pressure, and subsequently diabetes as well among the people that I worked with in Cairo. "This is why it's important to laugh a lot and not think too much," Ahmed argues above. Ahmed was not the only person I met in Cairo to mention laughter in relation to the notion of *ḍaghṭ*, both as a way to relieve the pressures of everyday life and as a way to ease one's blood pressure (in the following chapter I will unfold how the notion of *ḍaghṭ* is also used to refer to the pathological condition of hypertension). In fact, it is common in Egypt to refer to a person who is humorous and lighthearted by nature by saying, "*Huwa ʿindo dam khafīf*," which literally means, "He has light-weighted blood." In other words, if you are prone to laughter, your blood will flow more easily and the *ḍaghṭ*, or pressures, of everyday life will be released more easily as well. However, as depicted throughout the above, laughter carries more than potential relief as it may also generate uncertainty and tension.

In this chapter, I have argued that humor and laughter provided the people I came across in Cairo with a common space of communication without succumbing to the certainty of specific narratives or so-called facts. Humor and laughter were drawn upon as a way to resist, for example, harmful and unnecessary medical treatment; however, the presence of humor and laughter also left people in a state of great uncertainty as to how to move forward in many spheres of everyday life, including in relation to medical advice.

I will end this chapter with one final reversal, a rendition of yet another satirical cartoon picturing what appears to be President al-Sisi (although, once again, he is not named directly) in what I suspect many Egyptians would consider an unlikely situation of questioning the grounds of his own understandings and convictions. The cartoon was drawn by Andeel and first published on Madamasr.com in September of 2016. The cartoon was entitled "Existential president" and depicts the back of President al-Sisi, watching a Cairo night skyline, contemplating in a thought bubble, "*ʾAkīd ʾanā ṣaḥ … ṣaḥ?!* Surely I am right … right?!" The cartoon illustrates the sentiment of uncertainty and ambiguity that prevailed throughout many spheres of everyday life in Cairo throughout my fieldwork in the years of 2015–2017; the Egyptian word *ṣaḥ* used in the above more directly translated into English as "true" rather than "right," indicating a beholder of the "truth" or the most accurate rendition of reality.

In this chapter, I have aimed to illustrate how the fundamental question of "What is true?" characterized various spheres of everyday life in Cairo, and how this question was rarely resolved with definite answers; rather, doubt and uncertainties lingered as an intrinsic part of everyday life, both in medical and in social spheres. In the following chapter, I will unfold how the question of "What is true?" manifested particularly in relation to type-2 diabetes. In the following chapters, I will move on to unfold the subsequent question of "What to do?" in relation to the treatment of the condition.

Notes

1 One of the wealthier neighborhoods in Cairo.
2 Parts of this ethnographic vignette have previously been published in the book chapter, "Risky Notes" (see Thorsen 2020).

References

Asad, Talal. 2012. Fear and the Ruptured State: Reflections on Egypt after Mubarak. *Social Research* 79(2): 271–298.

Bergson, Henri. 1911. *Laughter: An Essay on the Meaning of the Comic*. Macmillan.

Cameron, William Bruce. 1963. *Informal Sociology*. Random House.

Carty, John, and Yasmine Musharbash. 2008. You've Got to Be Joking: Asserting the Analytical Value of Humour and Laughter in Contemporary Anthropology. *Anthropological Forum* 18(3): 209–217.

Douglas, Mary. 1966. *Purity and Danger*. Routledge.

El-Ghobashy, Mona. 2021. *Bread and Freedom: Egypt's Revolutionary Situation*. Stanford University Press.

Ewing, Katherine P. 1990. The Illusion of Wholeness: Culture, Self, and the Experience of Inconsistency. *Ethos* 18(3): 251–278.

Ghannam, Farha. 2013. *Live and Die Like a Man: Gender Dynamics in Urban Egypt*. Stanford University Press.

Goldstein, Donna. 2003. *Laughter Out of Place: Race, Class, Violence and Sexuality in a Brazilian Favela*. University of California Press.

Green, Linda. 1994. Fear as a Way of Life. *Cultural Anthropology* 9(2): 227–256.

Hamdy, Sherine F. 2012. *Our Bodies Belong to God: Organ Transplants, Islam, and the Struggle for Human Dignity in Egypt*. University of California Press.

Hamdy, Sherine F., and Soha Bayoumi. 2016. Egypt's Popular Uprising and the Stakes of Medical Neutrality. *Culture, Medicine, and Psychiatry* 40(2): 223–241.

Helmy, Mohamed M., and Sabine Frerichs. 2013. Stripping the Boss: The Powerful Role of Humor in the Egyptian Revolution 2011. *Integrative Psychological and Behavioral Science* 47(4): 450–481.

Inhorn, Marcia C. 1994. *Quest for Conception: Gender, Infertility and Egyptian Medical Traditions*. University of Pennsylvania Press.

Jackson, Michael. 2002. *The Politics of Storytelling: Violence, Transgression, and Intersubjectivity*. University of Chicago Press.

Keisalo, Marianna. 2016. "Picking People to Hate": Reversible Reversals in Stand-up Comedy. *Suomen Antropologi: Journal of the Finnish Anthropological Society* 41(4): 62–76.

Keisalo, Marianna. 2018. Perspectives of (and on) a Comedic Self: A Semiotics of Subjectivity in Stand-up Comedy. *Social Analysis* 62(1): 116–135.

Khachab, Chihab el. 2017. Compressing Scales: Characters and Situations in Egyptian Internet Humor. *Middle East Critique* 26(4): 331–353.

Malmström, Maria Frederika. 2019. *The Streets Are Talking to Me: Affective Fragments in Sisi's Egypt*. University of California Press.

Michaelson, Ruth. 2017. Egypt Blocks Access to News Websites Including Al-Jazeera and Mada Masr. May 25, 2017. The Guardian. www.theguardian.com/world/2017/may/25/egypt-blocks-access-news-websites-al-jazeera-mada-masr-press-freedom.

Mitchell, Timothy. 2002. *Rule of Experts: Egypt, Techno-Politics, Modernity*. University of California Press.

Norbakk, Mari. 2018. Men of Light Blood: Revolution Stories, Humor, and Masculine Capital in Egypt. *Men and Masculinities* 21(3): 328–340.

Pelkmans, Mathijs. 2013. *Ethnographies of Doubt: Faith and Uncertainty in Contemporary Societies*. I. B. Tauris.

Pelkmans, Mathijs. 2016. The Restlessness of Doubt, and the Tenacity of Belief. *HAU Journal of Ethnographic Theory* 6(1): 499–503.

Pierce, Charles S. 1998. *The Essential Writings*. Prometheus Books.

Proctor, Robert N. 2008. Agnotology: A Missing Term to Describe the Cultural Production of Ignorance (and Its Study). *In Agnotology: The Making and Unmaking of Ignorance*. Robert N. Proctor, and Londa Schiebinger, eds. Pp. 1–33. Stanford University Press.

Redmond, Anthony. 2008. Captain Cook Meets General Macarthur in the Northern Kimberley: Humour and Ritual in an Indigenous Australian Life-World. *Anthropological Forum* 18(3): 255–270.

Schielke, Samuli J. 2009. Ambivalent Commitments: Troubles of Morality, Religiosity and Aspiration among Young Egyptians. *Journal of Religion in Africa* 39(2): 158–185.

Scott, James C. 1985. *Weapons of the Weak: Everyday Forms of Peasant Resistance*. Yale University Press.

Shehata, Samer S. 1992. The Politics of Laughter: Nasser, Sadat, and Mubarek in Egyptian Political Jokes. *Folklore* 103(1): 75–91.

Thorsen, Mille K. 2020. Risky Notes: Reading Tense Situations in Cairo in 2015. *In Anthropology Inside Out: Fieldworkers Taking Note*. A. Andersen, L. Dalsgård, M. L. Kusk, et al., eds. Pp. 135–150. Sean Kingston Publishing.

Weems, Scott. 2014. *HA! The Science of When We Laugh and Why*. Basic Books.

Zijderveld, Anton C. 1983. Introduction: The Sociology of Humour and Laughter – An Outstanding Debt. *Current Sociology* 33(3): 1–6.

3 Food[1]

International medical guidelines and research on the treatment of type-2 diabetes recount a condition with the potential to spiral out of control, and thus articulate treatment largely as a matter of "controlling" the illness (see, for example, Barnard et al. 2018; Farag and Gaballa 2011; Kalra et al. 2013; WHO 2016); a rhetoric and approach promoted also by doctors and other healthcare personnel throughout my research in Cairo. This was evident, for example, in the encouragement by doctors and others of patients to monitor and control blood sugars, calories, and weight by means of medications, diet plans, and exercise. This approach to treatment was apparent also in the abundance of brochures often printed by multinational medical companies and distributed to people with type-2 diabetes across various healthcare facilities in Cairo, including brochures meant to assist patients with keeping food diaries and blood sugar diaries, as well as pamphlets containing general dietary guidelines.

The specific idea of controlling the body through certain actions (such as exercising and dieting) can be traced back to ancient Greece. Historian Shigehisa Kuriyama has outlined how ancient Greek physicians viewed the body as made primarily of muscle, but muscle that could be trained and brought under control. This, Kuriyama argues, subsequently shaped a perspective of the subject as potentially in control of the body (Kuriyama 1999:111–51). Philosopher Annemarie Mol draws inspiration from these arguments in her work on diabetes care in the Netherlands when outlining how "citizens," not "patients," are expected to control and postpone bodily needs and urges, even when diagnosed with diabetes (Mol 2008a; Mol 2008b). In this chapter, I will show how a neoliberal responsibilization of the individual in relation to type-2 diabetes – drawing on the above specific understandings of subjects potentially in control of their bodies – was largely drawn upon by healthcare professionals

DOI: 10.4324/9781003327684-3

in Cairo in their particular and persistent foregrounding of the relation of obesity to type-2 diabetes. However, among the families that I worked with, and among the hundreds of patients I encountered across various healthcare facilities, obesity did not seem to play a significant role in relation to the onset or condition of type-2 diabetes. Rather, "*ḍaghṭ*," loosely translated as "stress," more literally as "pressure," was believed to cause the condition.

In the first part of this chapter, I explore the notion of *ḍaghṭ*, and how it was referred to by people in Cairo in many spheres of everyday life. Particularly, I argue that understandings of *ḍaghṭ*, when related to the onset of type-2 diabetes, essentially placed the condition first in the environment, then in the body. Thus, many of the people that I worked with in Cairo who were diagnosed with type-2 diabetes expressed that it was their surroundings that needed to be controlled and managed, rather than the self as such.

In the subsequent parts of the chapter, I explore these arguments in relation to the specific topic of food and beverage intake. I recount how common dietary advice given by doctors and other healthcare professionals in Cairo was rarely put to use by people living with type-2 diabetes, as they did not consider their weight or nutrition to be relevant to their diabetic condition as such. However, the price, quality, and availability of food and beverages were closely linked to the notion of *ḍaghṭ* and thus to the onset and general condition of type-2 diabetes.

From this perspective, food and beverage intake did matter in relation to type-2 diabetes to those in Cairo who were living with the condition. However, this was not considered in relation to the number of calories or composition of nutrients consumed, but rather in relation to political and environmental factors affecting the prices, availability, and quality of food and beverages. I will illustrate how uncertainties regarding the environment (for example, in relation to shifting economies and food prices) were intrinsic to the notion of *ḍaghṭ* and thus also to the condition of type-2 diabetes. In other words, although people in Cairo displayed firm beliefs about the relation of *ḍaghṭ* to type-2 diabetes, these beliefs were still constituted by uncertainties in relation to a range of aspects of everyday life, including uncertainties as to how these aspects potentially affected bodies and beings.

In the final part of the chapter, I will unfold the specific case of a sugar shortage that happened across Egypt in the fall of 2016, and how people in Cairo were relating this shortage to notions of *ḍaghṭ* and type-2 diabetes specifically. I will draw on this particular case to discuss how understandings of type-2 diabetes have commonly been linked to matters of abundance and affluence, both within biomedical literature and in common rhetoric, for example, in Europe and North America. However, among those I worked with in Cairo who were diagnosed with type-2 diabetes, shortages of food, including the shortage of sugar, were rather seen as related to the onset and condition of type-2 diabetes. As opposed to linking type-2 diabetes to matters of abundance and affluence, the condition was, in other words, more commonly linked to matters of deprivation and scarcity, and more specifically to the experiences of *ḍaghṭ* brought on by such potential deprivation and scarcity.

The Kitchen (May 2015)

I am sitting with Maha at her mother-in-law's house. Maha sits on the floor with legs stretched out in front of her, her feet swollen from her pregnancy and the hot weather. She is lost in her thoughts. Her mother-in-law is stretched out on the couch, watching a cooking show on TV, with the remote control in one hand and her cell phone in the other. On TV a woman is cooking burgers and a chocolate cake.

"There is a lot of fruit on the plate. That's good. It's healthy," Maha's mother-in-law says. Neither Maha nor I reply.

I stare at the aquariums that surround the TV. The aquariums are large, with several turtles swimming around inside them. Maha's father-in-law comes up the stairs with a bag of oranges. "Why are you on the floor?" he asks Maha.

"So I can stretch my legs out like this," Maha says, covering her swollen feet with her dress. "The doctor says it's good for me." Maha's father-in-law does not respond, but leaves the bag of oranges on the kitchen counter, and goes to the balcony.

Maha gets up and I follow her into the kitchen; she begins cutting the oranges and prepares to make juice. I sit on a low chair, curled up in the corner of the kitchen. I catch and crush a small cockroach with my hands. I try to wipe my hands with a tissue as I ask Maha about her mother-in-law's diabetes.

Maha stops cutting the oranges for a while; a look of concentration creeps across her face as she tries to remember. "I think she got it six years ago. The neighbor's apartment burnt down." Maha points toward the small kitchen window with the knife still in her hand.

I get up to wash my hands and look out the window. I see many buildings, and wonder which one she is talking about.

"Her neighbor was still inside," Maha continues. "She heard him screaming. He was burnt alive. She got diabetes from *il-khaḍḍa*, the shock."

I look at Maha, a bit shocked myself. I dry my hands and return to my chair in the corner, asking Maha how exactly her mother-in-law got diabetes from "*il-khaḍḍa*, the shock."

"The shock affects the pressure, *il-ḍaghṭ*, somehow. I don't know how exactly. But *il-ḍaghṭ* gave her diabetes," Maha says.

I sit in silence for a while as Maha rummages through the cupboards. I ask how her mother-in-law first noticed her diabetes.

Maha returns to cutting the oranges. She tells me, "Well, first she retired from her job, then she gained a lot of weight because she would just sit at home and eat. *Like now*," Maha whispers, with a quiet laugh. "But she gained maybe 20 kilos, and then suddenly she lost a lot of weight, even though she wasn't on a diet," Maha explains, as she eats an orange slice. "So she went to the doctor, and the doctor told her that she had a lot of sugar in her blood, *sukkar kathīr fī il-dam*." Maha begins pressing the juice. "She is always very tired from her diabetes. Her body is always causing her pain."

Maha hands me a glass of juice, and I thank her after taking a refreshing sip. "My mother-in-law can be very nervous, *ʿaṣabīya*. My father-in-law is the opposite, very calm, *ḥadiʾ*. That's why my mother-in-law is more ill than he is," Maha says. "Because being so nervous affects the blood pressure, *il-ḍaghṭ*."

Maha arranges the glasses on a tray, and we return to the living room where she serves her mother-in-law a glass of the freshly squeezed juice. She thanks Maha and goes back to watching an episode of an Egyptian soap opera. I sit down and try to engage in the soap opera as well. We watch together as a girl in her 20s enters a living room; the girl's mother sits on the couch while peeling vegetables, and the girl yawns while saying "good morning" as she sits down next to her mother.

"Good morning? It's noon! Why do you always sleep in so late?" the mother asks.

"Do we have to have this same conversation every morning?" the girl responds. "Why should I get up early? What should I do? Speak to myself? *Baba* buys all the groceries and you do all the work in the house. What am I supposed to do?"

"You should look for a husband!" the mother promptly responds.

Both Maha and her mother-in-law burst out laughing. Maha turns to me and says, "It is like this in all Egyptian families. There is always pressure, *ḍaghṭ*, for the girl to find a husband." Maha's mother-in-law nods in agreement. The girl and her mother in the soap opera quickly end their conversation. "*Insha'allah*, God willing," the girl will soon find a husband.

The Cause of Diabetes (Introducing Maha)

When I first arrived in Cairo in 2015 for my initial phase of fieldwork, I stayed with a young woman, Maha, and her family in a small town north of Cairo. Before my arrival, Maha had recently married Mustafa and was pregnant with their first child. (Maha and Mustafa were first cousins, and so Maha's mother-in-law was also her maternal aunt.) The couple lived in their own apartment, down the street from the house of Mustafa's parents – most of their family lived within walking distance in the same neighborhood. During my nearly two-month stay with the family, Maha was working as an Arabic teacher in the public school down the street, as well as teaching private classes online. Mustafa worked as an advertiser for a public newspaper in downtown Cairo. Their parents were all retired and living off their pensions and savings. Maha's mother, mother-in-law, maternal grandmother, and several of her aunts and uncles (both maternal and paternal) were diagnosed with type-2 diabetes; Maha's father was also diagnosed with type-2 diabetes, but had passed away in 2013 shortly after having also been diagnosed with liver cancer. Maha's mother-in-law was especially ill from her diabetes during my stay with the family, and Maha would often step in to help her with everyday chores, such as cleaning the house, shopping for groceries, and cooking meals.

Across the different families that I worked with in Cairo, as well as among the majority of the patients that I observed in various healthcare facilities in the city, I frequently experienced people relating their type-2 diabetes to the notion of *ḍaghṭ*. Loosely translated, my English-speaking Egyptian friends would translate *ḍaghṭ* as "stress." When asked to elaborate further, they gave me the literal English translation of "pressure," with most people placing their hands on top of their heads to illustrate *ḍaghṭ* as something heavy, weighing them down. This is perhaps a clear indication that "pressure" is a more accurate, or at least more literal, translation of *ḍaghṭ* than "stress."

The English use of the term "stress" tends to put an emphasis on temporality, a period of time when one is busy or rushed (see, for example, Flaherty 2011; and Funahashi 2013), whereas the Egyptian *ḍaghṭ* tends to emphasize volume over temporality. Something is causing a pressure, and this pressure is weighing people down and pushing them around. The notion of *ḍaghṭ* is also used by Egyptian healthcare professionals and laymen alike to refer to one's blood pressure, as well as to the specific condition of hypertension (high blood pressure). The people that I met in Cairo who suffered from hypertension would thus simply say, " *'indī ḍaghṭ*," meaning literally that "I have pressure," or, more accurately translated, that "I suffer from high blood pressure." In this sense, the notion of *ḍaghṭ* also offered a temporal dimension, a potential to either rush or slow down the circulation of blood.

The use of the Egyptian *ḍaghṭ* has many parallels to the English use of the term "stress," in the sense that both tend to cover an infinite number of stimuli external to the body as well as various physiological responses within the body (see, for example, Charlton 1992; and Young 1980 for early critical reviews of such uses of the term "stress"). Physician Hans Selye, who was a pioneer in outlining the notion of stress, summed up its all-encompassing ability as "the nonspecific response of the body to any demand" (Selye 1976:53). Today, the English notion of stress holds both a pathological diagnosis and a subjective experience of suffering (what anthropologist Arthur Kleinman would differentiate respectively as "disease" and "illness"; see Kleinman 1980). This also applies to the Egyptian *ḍaghṭ*, though the pathological diagnosis here is hypertension specifically, rather than a separate category of stress as such.

Returning to Maha and others from my fieldwork in Cairo, most of them referred to something or someone as causing *ḍaghṭ kathīr*, "a lot of pressure." As is the case with the English term "stress," the Egyptian *ḍaghṭ* was rather unspecified; it included both emotional and physiological pressures and it referred to both specifics and abstractions (paralleling, in many ways, anthropologist Byron Good's arguments of "heart distress" in 1970s Iran; see Good 1977). Some of the factors seen by Maha and others as causing *ḍaghṭ* included: pollution, heat, dust, transportation, traffic, exams, inflation, elections, bureaucracies, hospitals, police, weddings, engagements, husbands, wives, mothers, mother-in-laws, and the Cairene crowds in general – or, as Maha described earlier, traumatic events and the expectations of women (and men) to find a suitable spouse.

Anthropologist Mohammed Tabishat has argued that these aspects of *ḍaghṭ* are exactly why it has become such a household term in Cairo, "For large numbers of the Cairene population *al-daght* is one concept that is readily communicable and an illness that is easy to contract" (Tabishat 2000:203). When drawing on the expression of *ḍaghṭ*, Maha and others instantly related environmental and social factors to physiological ones. As Ahmed, the gardener, stated toward the end of the previous chapter, "Pressure from life, *ḍaghṭ min il-ḥayā*, will result in a pressure in your blood, *ḍaghṭ fī il-dam*." Put differently, the countless pressures or stress factors of living in Cairo, so Maha, Ahmed, and others argued, affected their blood pressure over time. This, they further argued, potentially caused type-2 diabetes. Type-2 diabetes was thus placed, first, in the environment, and, then, in the body.

Biomedical research does indeed relate the condition of stress to type-2 diabetes. Physiologically, stress drives the body to mobilize a great amount of energy as is evident, for example, in an increase of sugars and fats in the blood, as well as an increase in the blood pressure. Such stress reactions occur frequently in all humans, but if the reactions are prolonged, and the body does not get to restitute, the stress will eventually turn harmful. Prolonged stress reactions may cause deleterious changes, for example, to the cardiovascular, metabolic, and immune systems, potentially causing an onset of, for example, type-2 diabetes (see, for example, Corazon et al. 2010; Nielsen et al. 2008; Tsiotra and Tsigos 2006).

Even though biomedical research does relate stress to type-2 diabetes, this etiology is often de-emphasized within biomedical literature in favor of an etiology of "diabesity." However, relating type-2 diabetes to emotions such as pressure or stress is not unique to people in Egypt at all. Anthropological literature from many different ethnographic settings thus recounts similar stories as the ones I encountered in Egypt. Broom and Whittaker, for example, have outlined how Australians relate "stress" to the onset of diabetes (Broom and Whittaker 2004:2375–6); a range of social scientists have outlined how Mexicans and Mexican-Americans tend to relate the Spanish "susto," fright, and "nervios," nerves, or the English "stress," to the onset of diabetes (see, for example, Baer et al. 2012; Schoenberg et al. 2005; Seligman et al. 2015); Rock has outlined how Aboriginal populations in Canada relate "mental distress" and "suffering" to the onset of diabetes (Rock 2003); Qureshi mentions "worries" as related to diabetes among Pakistani women in Britain (Qureshi 2013); and finally, Little, Humphries, Patel, and Dewey (Little et al. 2017), as well as Solomon (Solomon 2016) and Weaver (Weaver 2018), all outline the English-Hindi notion of "tenshun," tension, as being related to the onset of diabetes by people in India.

Several social scientists have discussed on a more general level the porosity of the body to the environment in similar ways as captured by the notion of *ḍaghṭ* (see, for example, Ingold 2000; Leder 1990; Mol 2008b). From his work on diabetes in Mumbai, anthropologist

Harris Solomon has, for example, outlined the notion of "metabolic living" as a way to capture the intermingling of bodies, environments, and substances in relation to the condition of diabetes specifically. Drawing on this particular conceptualization, he raises the fundamental questions, "Who and what become the eater and the eaten? What is nutrition and what is poison? Who and what set the boundaries of inside and outside, delineating organism and environment?" (Solomon 2016:5).

Maha and others raised similar questions in relation to the interaction of their bodies with their environment, and how such interaction potentially caused ailments such as type-2 diabetes. From the perspective of Maha and others, it was the surroundings that needed to be controlled and managed in relation to type-2 diabetes, not the self or the body as such. Diabetes treatment thus rarely came to revolve around those diagnosed with type-2 diabetes measuring their blood sugars on a regular basis (this was usually done once a year in relation to visits to the doctor's – an exception is found in the following chapter as Taher, a young doctor, measured his mother's blood sugar on a weekly basis). It was neither carried out by counting calories, engaging in physical exercise, or attempting to lose weight. Rather, diabetes treatment came to revolve primarily around ways of relieving the ill of pressures, *ḍaghṭ*, induced by factors in the surroundings. In the following, I will elaborate on this understanding of Maha and others by zooming in on the topic of food in relation to type-2 diabetes specifically.

The Doctor's Office (May 2015)

I wait in the car with Maha and her mother, while Abdullah (Maha's younger brother) picks up their mother's lab results. He quickly returns and hands Maha the results. He sees me examining their old, worn-down car. "Like a tuktuk, only closed," he says in Arabic with a laugh. I smile.

Maha examines their mother's lab results and then hands me the paper. "What do you think? Do the results look normal to you?" Maha and her mother both look at me as I scan the results, but I tell them that I really do not know.

The car makes a loud cracking sound as Abdullah tries to start the engine. It nearly lurches down the street as he finally starts the motor. Light pours out from streetside shops as the evening grows darker. The car has no headlights. Everyone seems to be honking at us. I wonder if Abdullah has a driver's license. After all, he is only 17.

Abdullah remains focused as he drives. The car stalls when we hit a traffic jam. Maha looks patiently at Abdullah as he scrambles to get the car moving again. Some young boys in a tuktuk stop and cheer for Abdullah when he successfully reignites the engine. Everyone but Abdullah laughs, and we all wave at each other.

Abdullah decides to take the backroads, "away from traffic," he comments. We pass a large landfill, and I watch as some men bring their sheep to graze in the garbage.

We finally make it to the right street and park the car along the sidewalk. I step out of the car with Maha and her mother and we enter an apartment building. "The doctor's office is on the third floor," Maha says, and we slowly climb the stairs together.

A nurse sits at the front desk, and Maha tells me in a hushed voice that we have to give her some money, "a tip," otherwise we will be waiting all night. I look around at the waiting room, which is completely empty. Maha discretely gives the nurse some money and asks where the doctor is. "She is praying," the nurse responds. Maha decides to pray as well, and goes by herself into a backroom, returning after a short while. The nurse then quickly shows us to the doctor's office.

The doctor seems similar in age to Maha's mother. She gives us a friendly smile as she reaches for the lab results. The doctor runs her pen down the paper and says, "It's better than last time, but it's still not good." The doctor starts explaining that she suspects Maha's mother is not "eating correctly." Maha's mother argues that her problem is not what she eats, but that she has been feeling sad since her husband passed away almost two years ago. "My blood sugar is too high *min il-zaʿil*, from the sadness, and because of *il-ḍaghṭ*, the pressure from the sadness," she says.

The doctor looks at Maha's mother, shakes her head and says, "*Lā, min il-ʾakl*, no, it's from the food." The doctor then measures Maha's mother's blood pressure. After a while, she looks at Maha's mother and comments, "Look, *ya Mama*, your blood pressure, *ḍaghṭik*, it's fine."

The doctor starts asking Maha's mother about her diet. Instead of responding to the doctor's questions, Maha's mother starts asking questions of her own.

"Is it okay to eat falafel?" she asks.

"Falafel is really bad when you have diabetes!" the doctor says. We all laugh. Maha's mother asks a couple of other questions about food. The doctor interrupts and asks how much tea Maha's mother drinks during the day? Maha quickly responds, "5 to 6 cups!" Her mother responds a second too late, "1 to 2 cups." The two of them look at each other and start laughing. The doctor then asks how many teaspoons of sugar Maha's mother puts in her tea. Maha is quick again, "2 to 3 teaspoons," while her mother says, "1 teaspoon." The doctor looks at the two women, dramatically mimicking great disbelief. We all laugh.

The doctor then tells Maha's mother that she is definitely not allowed to drink that much sugar in her tea. The doctor begins listing which fruits are especially "*mamnūʿ*, forbidden" when you have diabetes. Mangos. Figs. Dates. Grapes. Maha's mother starts discussing the different fruits with the doctor. She has heard that figs are good when you have diabetes.

"Where did you hear that? From a doctor or from a friend?" the doctor asks. Maha and her mother laugh again.

"What about pomegranate?" Maha's mother then asks.

"NO!" The doctor yells. We all laugh. Maha's mother grumbles that she likes to eat *a lot* of pomegranate. The doctor suggests that Maha's mother visit a dietitian. She finally ends the consultation, "*Khalāṣ*, alright, *ya Mama*."

We make our way down the stairs and return to the street to find Abdullah waiting for us; we pile into the car, but the car won't start. "You are kidding, right?" Maha says, as if Abdullah has purposely broken the car while we were away. A tuktuk passes us as we try to get the car started again, and I suggest that we ask the tuktuk driver to help us push the car; Abdullah calls out to the driver, who graciously decides to help us. Maha's mother sits in the car while Maha, the tuktuk driver, and I push the car until Abdullah finally gets the engine running again. Maha complains about her swollen feet and pregnant belly as we jog alongside the car and jump into the backseat. We slam the doors of the rolling car, laughing hysterically.

Maha's mother immediately turns around and suggests that we get ice cream. *Mango* ice cream. "Two things I am not allowed to eat," she says with a laugh. Maha laughs as well, before yelling in a scolding voice, "*Ya MAMA!*"

The Management of Diabetes

Among the people I was working with in Cairo who were diagnosed with type-2 diabetes, most would see an endocrinologist (hormone specialist) once a year. Most attended a private clinic, such as Maha's mother; others would visit an outpatient clinic at one of the public hospitals in Cairo. I observed hundreds of doctors' consultations during my research in Cairo, during which the majority of patients were told by their doctors that their blood sugar levels were too high. In the words of the doctors, the blood sugar levels were "*mish maṣbūṭ*, not precise" or "not right" (that is, poorly regulated). While some doctors would try to change their patients' medications, most would put greater emphasis on weight loss and better nutrition. As in the above example with Maha's mother, this especially revolved around listing which foods were considered "*mamnūʿ*, forbidden," for someone diagnosed with type-2 diabetes.

However, similar to Maha's mother, most of the people that I knew well in Cairo who were diagnosed with type-2 diabetes, as well as patients that I observed more briefly during various doctors' consultations, had different understandings as to why their blood sugar was poorly regulated than the reasons given by their doctors. Rather than relating their poorly regulated blood sugars to the intake of "forbidden" foods and beverages, or to the intake of too many calories in general, Maha's mother and others would mention emotions such as *zaʿil*, "sadness," *ʿaṣabīya*, "nervousness," *khawf*, "fear," and *iktiʾāb*, "depression," as causing *ḍaghṭ*, pressure, and thus literally as affecting their blood pressure and their condition of type-2 diabetes as well (see also Tabishat 2000 for similar accounts of the relation of *ḍaghṭ* to a range of emotions). As was the case with Maha's mother, it was common for doctors to point to the fact that, often, the patient did not actually suffer from the condition of *ḍaghṭ* in a pathological sense; that is, from high blood pressure.

The dietary advice given by doctors in Egypt to patients with type-2 diabetes corresponds with that which is outlined in current biomedical research on the subject (see, for example, Gray 2015 for a literature review on nutritional recommendations for individuals with diabetes). In short, the dietary guidelines during medical consultations in Cairo were given for two primary reasons: to encourage weight loss among those who were considered to be overweight (which was the case of most patients), and to avoid high fluctuations in blood sugar levels, which could cause late-stage complications (such as cardiovascular disease, stroke, kidney failure, blindness, and amputations). The advice given by the Egyptian doctors outlined how half a plate of food should contain vegetables, a quarter of a plate of lean meat and a quarter of a plate of whole-grains (such as brown rice), while avoiding the use of ghee/clarified butter when cooking. Fruit was allowed, but only those with the lowest concentration of fructose, such as apples, strawberries, oranges, and peaches. Doctors also advised against soft drinks, juice, tea, and coffee in general, due to the potentially high intake of added or natural sugars in these beverages.

Comparing some of these dietary guidelines with the diet in most of the homes that I visited in Cairo, the majority of main meals contained at least two or three carbohydrates, such as white rice, bread, fried potatoes, couscous, and/or pasta. This often constituted more than a quarter of the food on the plate (if not the majority of the meal). In addition, apart from the bread, which was usually bought at local bakeries, all these carbohydrates were cooked in ghee and cooking oil before being boiled in water. Along with these carbs, a small bowl of fresh greens was often served, primarily tomatoes, cucumber, and lettuce. Other greens such as eggplant, cabbage, and zucchini were cooked with the meat and sauce, as were beans and lentils. Chicken, pigeon, and duck were the most common meat, but also lamb and beef. In fact, a few of the families, including Maha's family, bred their own poultry on the roof of their buildings.

In the summer, it was often difficult to buy fresh vegetables apart from the ones mentioned above. Rather, there was an abundance of fruit, fresh and dried, such as mangos, melons, grapes, dates, pomegranates, and figs. Fruits were served as a snack and as juices and smoothies. Most of these beverages were spiked with sugar, as was the tea and coffee. Snacking at Maha's house rarely revolved around the intake of sweets such as candy, cake, and ice cream, but rather around the intake of fruit and mixed nuts, as well as juices, tea, and coffee (all spiked with plenty of sugar). To illustrate the importance of some of the above food items, I might mention here that the Egyptian government subsidizes sugar, cooking oil, white rice, wheat pasta, and bread, allowing for most families to access these particular goods at affordable prices.

Despite a reluctance to accept calories and nutrients as directly related to their type-2 diabetes, Maha's mother and others did attempt to integrate some of the advice given by their doctors in relation to their eating habits. Maha's mother and mother-in-law, for example, made sure to only eat one type of carb with their lunch and dinner (instead of having, for example, both rice, potatoes, and bread), and Maha's mother-in-law would only use artificial sweetener in her tea instead of regular sugar. Other dietary advice was not so easily accepted. This was, for example, the case especially of advice countering the advice of prophetic medicine (Sheikh 2016). Dates, for example, are renowned in Egypt for their many healthy qualities and are mentioned as such in several places in the Qur'an and in Hadiths of the Prophet. Breaking the fast during Ramadan, for example, should be done by eating a date, as did the Prophet.

Dates were also believed to ease the pain of labor during childbirth, and if eaten during pregnancy they were additionally believed by many to give the mother an "intelligent" child. In summary, no one within the families that I worked with in Cairo was willing to accept the fact that dates were suddenly "forbidden" and somehow considered unhealthy. I might add here that none of the people I worked with in Cairo who were diagnosed with type-2 diabetes were preoccupied specifically with foods believed within prophetic medicine to be particularly useful in relation to type-2 diabetes; rather such foods were considered in general to be good for one's health and wellbeing. In addition to dates, I might mention here honey and figs as well.

The above dietary adjustments of Maha's mother and mother-in-law more or less covered the extent to which the above-outlined dietary advice manifested in the lives of people within the families that I worked with the closest. Overall, I did not speak to anyone in Cairo who had tried to lose weight on the grounds of having been diagnosed with type-2 diabetes. Weight, calories, and nutrients thus simply did not play a significant role in relation to type-2 diabetes in the minds of most of these people, contrary to the understandings and advice given by their doctors. In fact, most of those I spoke with in general on the topic of obesity believed that some degree of overweight (by BMI standards, see, for example, Long et al. 1998) was a sign of health (and beauty). Thus, I only ever heard a few young women discuss overweight as a health issue, whereas I heard many other people of all ages and both genders discuss women, in particular, who were considered too skinny to be healthy (for example, to bear a child). To be clear, categories of overweight, or of being "fat, *takhīn*," do exist in Egypt, but the definition differs greatly from the medical BMI standards and even then overweight is rarely considered a negative label of, for example, an unhealthy body. Anthropological work from within Egypt has discussed an increasing adoption of skinnier body ideals, particularly among younger generations within the wealthier segments of society (see, for example, Basyouny 1998; Ghannam and Sholkamy 2004). This was, however, not yet evident among the people I worked with in Cairo.

Anthropologist Deborah Lupton has previously discussed the "moralizing" aspects of "fatness" particularly evident in parts of Europe and North America. Lupton outlines how being overweight in these parts of the world is often perceived as matters of "gluttony" or "deviant and uncontrolled physical practices" (Lupton 2013:51). Anthropologist Gareth Williams has similarly argued on a more general note that the understanding of health in Europe and North America has been presented throughout history "as a matter of right conduct" whereas "illness is a sign of sinfulness" (Williams 2002:92). This is evident also in relation to present-day understandings of type-2 diabetes, often termed in parts of Europe and North America as a "lifestyle disease," and its treatment a matter of "lifestyle choices" (see, for example, Ferzacca 2012; Mol 2008a; and Rock 2003 for critical studies on the implications of such understandings for people diagnosed with type-2 diabetes). Recent literature within the field of anthropology has critically examined this neoliberal understanding and individual responsibilization of a range of health issues, including type-2 diabetes. This literature argues that a neoliberal understanding of type-2 diabetes has resulted in a foregrounding of risk factors such as obesity above other known risk factors related, for example, to structural and political issues. Likewise, the responsibilization of obesity has similarly been placed within the moral realm of the individual, rather than within a structural or political framework (see, for example, Glasgow and Schrecker 2016; Phillips, McMichael, and O'Keefe 2018; Reubi, Herrick, and Brown 2016; and Trnka and Trundle 2017).

Among the people I worked with in Cairo who were living with the condition, the understanding of *ḍaghṭ* as closely linked to type-2 diabetes placed the moral responsibility of their health primarily in their surroundings, not within their individual selves as such. Rather than being considered a result of "deviant" or "uncontrolled" behavior of the individual, as often conceptualized within a neoliberal context and prevailing among healthcare providers in Cairo as well, type-2 diabetes was linked by those diagnosed with the condition to an understanding of the surroundings as being fundamentally out-of-control, subsequently causing the body to be out-of-control with diabetes as well. Managing type-2 diabetes thus became a matter of shielding the individual diagnosed with diabetes from factors in the surroundings that might cause experiences of *ḍaghṭ*, as well as relieving existing *ḍaghṭ*. This was primarily done through various means of "resting, *istirāḥa*." In fact, "*istirāḥa*" was mentioned among all of the families that I worked with as the number one way to manage type-2 diabetes. Contrary to advice given by healthcare professionals to stay physically active, this meant that most of those who were diagnosed with the condition refrained from activities that might cause them any kind of physical strain. It also meant, for example, drinking lots of black tea with sugar, as this was known among everyone for its calming effects.

As evident throughout the above, global understandings of type-2 diabetes as related to obesity did not simply flow freely during medical consultations, but transformed through the streets of Cairo, manifesting, for example, in the way that the intake of foods and beverages was not considered to cause the onset of type-2 diabetes, or to affect the condition onwards, among those diagnosed with the condition, in the ways presented by healthcare personnel (and resembling those of international medical guidelines). However, it was considered an important factor both in relation to the onset and condition of type-2 diabetes, albeit in very different ways.

The Outdoor Market (May 2015)

I glance around the busy market; it is midday and burning hot. Maha is buying bananas from an old woman. The woman sits cross-legged on the ground. I hear Maha commenting on the bananas. "They are very small," she says to the woman. "But they are very good," the woman assures Maha. After a while Maha and the woman agree on a price. The woman uses an old-fashioned scale, adding and removing weights until she finally hands Maha the bananas in a plastic bag. Maha passes the bag on to me; it's very heavy.

We move along through the market. Slowly. Sweat runs down my face and back. Maha is shuffling from side to side, as if her back is aching. I look around at the large bins of vegetables and fruit for sale. The vegetables look squashed. The tomatoes look like they are almost boiling from the heat. The smell of decaying fruit and garbage is overwhelming. Flies cover basins of apricots and melons. I try to keep flies out of my nose and my eyes.

Maha is now buying some green beans, carefully selecting a handful from a huge pile, examining each bean closely before she hands them over to the woman selling them. A young woman interrupts and throws some of Maha's beans away. "They are rotten, look ...," she points. "These are better," she places a few other beans in Maha's hand. Maha argues with the bean seller about the price; apparently, the seller miscalculated. The young woman interferes again, taking Maha's side and arguing her case. The seller eventually gives in. Maha thanks the young stranger as we leave the bean vendor behind.

I look around the market. It's mostly full of women, balancing buckets of fruit and vegetables on their heads while trying to find the least squashed tomatoes and the least dried-out apricots. A young boy on a donkey makes a whistling noise at me as he rides by, and I jump aside. With all the activity, I try to stay close to

Maha. She is now arguing with a date seller about the price. She is sighing heavily in between her arguments. Sweat continues to drip down my face, and I feel layers of dirt sticking to it. I notice Maha wipes off sweat and dirt from her face with a tissue. She continues to hand me heavy bags of vegetables and fruit, as we slowly make our way through the market. Maha coughs and squints her eyes, as if the sun is hurting them. We pass by cages of live chickens and rabbits. There are droppings everywhere. Farther down the market, fresh fish is lying directly in the burning sun. The smell is awful.

Finally, we are ready to return to the house. Maha hails a tuktuk, and, with much difficulty, we mount it with all our bags. Maha sighs deeply. "My stomach hurts," she says in a low voice, as she caresses her pregnant belly. I tell her that we will be back at the house soon and she can then rest inside, out of the burning sun. "The house is really hot as well," she says, gazing out her side of the tuktuk.

Maha gives the address to the driver, and we set off. Shortly into the ride, the tuktuk hits a bump on the road. Maha snaps at the driver in an angry voice, "Careful!" The young tuktuk driver looks at us in the rear-view mirror; he picks up a chocolate bar and hands it to Maha. "For you," he says, glancing at her pregnant belly. Maha looks at him and says, "*Bil hanna*ʾ *wa il-shifā*ʾ, with pleasure and health, it's yours," politely refusing the gesture. We arrive at the house, and Maha instructs me to leave most of the groceries downstairs. "They are for Mustafa's mother," she sighs while pulling back her hijab and revealing the top of her head, hair drenched in sweat. She leaves the hijab hanging down her back, swaying from side to side, hands on her knees, as she slowly climbs the stairs to the apartment.

The Politics of Food

Maha and I frequented the market several times a week during my stay with her and her family. Most of our trips consisted of visits to the same specific vendors, where we would spend a substantial amount of time picking out the best products and arguing over the price. Upon returning from the market, and when dropping off the groceries at the house of Maha's mother-in-law, Maha and I would always be questioned about the groceries. "How much did you pay for the bananas?" "How much for the oranges?" "Did you go to the vendor in front of the flip flop shop or the one by the sponges and the soap?" "How much did you pay for the apricots?" "Look! This apricot is bad."

By the time of my second phase of fieldwork in Egypt in the spring of 2017, the economic crisis had deepened in the country due to the recent years of political turmoil (which had negatively affected the tourist sector and foreign investments). To counter the crisis, the Egyptian parliament took up a loan from the International Monetary Fund, but in order to meet key demands by the IMF in relation to the loan, the Egyptian pound was devalued by almost 50% (see, for example, Holodny 2016). This caused a great increase in the cost of almost everything. In some cases, food prices almost doubled. This naturally caused a great deal of strain on many of the families that I worked with in Cairo who were left prioritizing and minimizing their expenses.

In addition to prices increasing, and looming threats of various food shortages, Maha and others were also greatly concerned with the decreasing quality of food available at the time of my research. During the time of my fieldwork, families with a certain status of income could attain a ration card and use this card to buy state-subsidized goods, such as sugar, cooking oil, rice, pasta, and bread (approximately 80% of the Egyptian population has access to food by way of these ration cards; see, for example, LMC 2017:2). The card could be used only at certain shops, and only to attain the specific type of goods that were sold at these shops. The quality of the state-subsidized goods was frequently debated, also within Maha's family. "Look at the sugar. It's not even white. It looks dirty, *wasikh*," Maha told me at one point, speaking of a bag of state-subsidized sugar. "At the time of Mubarak, the sugar was white," she emphasized. "Look at the oil, it's almost black. How am I supposed to cook with this?" she also asked. "There are more pebbles than rice in this bag of rice. Look!"

Maha was generally concerned with the pollution of the food that was available to her, and which she had to cook and serve to her husband, his parents, and her pregnant self. She often discussed "*il-hurmūnāt*, the hormones," which she believed contaminated much of the food she bought at the market and at the state-subsidized shops as well. This was not exclusive to Maha. Maha's mother-in-law, for example, would never eat meat or egg from white chickens because white chickens were not considered "*balladi*, local." Rather, they were considered "*mustawrada*, imported" (even when born and bred down the street). Maha's mother-in-law would thus only eat meat and egg from the smaller, and more expensive, red chickens, as she believed this was better for her type-2 diabetes (see Hamdy 2008 for similar accounts in relation to the consumption of chicken in Egypt). During Maha's pregnancy, she would make an effort to eat more red chicken than white chicken, because, she argued, "It is better for the baby." At the peak of the financial crisis, this was not always possible due to the increasing prices and changes in availability, leaving Maha torn between eating the protein she knew to be good for the baby, and abstaining from eating meat that she thought to be potentially bad. Overall, from the perspective of Maha and others, shifts in the political landscape manifested as shifts in the quality of foods available as well.

Understandably, the price, availability, and quality of food were hot topics of conversation throughout my research stays in Egypt – and topics that seemed to go hand-in-hand with the state of affairs in the country. Going to the market, specifically, was in many ways an embodiment of the current state of affairs. For example, the ground which Maha had to cover to make whatever gains she set out to make changed simultaneously with the economy of the country. As prices spiked and food quality fell, she had to search the market – and sometimes her entire neighborhood and the city at large – to compare prices and qualities, and argue intensely with vendors (not only over price and quality, but also over loyalty, "I always buy my bananas from you!").

As evident in the ethnographic encounter above, leaving the house and enduring on a trip out in the city often meant enduring an intense sensory landscape of heat, dust, noise, traffic, and crowds. Consider, for example, how both Maha and I were consistently inhaling the dust from our surroundings. The dust stuck to our skin and in our throats and lungs. Walking under the midday sun burned our skin and drenched our clothes and hair with sweat. The physical and mental exhaustion of moving through the market, bargaining our way from vendor to vendor, was causing us first heavy breathing, then shallow breathing. And, finally, the exhaustion of moving from one vendor to the next was making our bodies ache, including a pregnant belly, knees, backs, and arms. The market place thus merged with our bodies and visibly affected our physical state of being. On returning from the market, Maha would, not surprisingly, often emphasize how the trip had been or had caused us "*ḍagḥṭ kathīr*, a lot of pressure."

Struggling to uphold certain standards of living put not only *ḍagḥṭ*, pressure, on, for example, Maha's pregnant body and her family's home economy, but also on her family relations. Maha was expected, for example, to acquire more or less the same goods from the market as before the inflation hit, and on more or less the same budget, despite the fact that prices had almost doubled. Both her mother-in-law and father-in-law would question her upon returning from the market, indicating (in Maha's perspective, anyway) that she had not put enough effort into bargaining or had gone to the wrong, and more expensive, vendors. Maha never argued with her in-laws, but she did release her frustrations on returning to her own house. She would often make comments such as, "She [her mother-in-law] forgot what it is like to go to the market. She never goes!" "She forgot how much *ḍaghṭ*, pressure, it can be to go to the market." "Does she not realize that everything costs more? It has nothing to do with me! It's the situation in the whole country."

Other families who took part in my research were also discussing how to prioritize their family budget in relation to the new economic situation. How much milk should the toddler drink, for example. This entanglement of the economy with the physiology of the body was also mirrored in a satirical cartoon by cartoonist Anwar published in the privately owned newspaper *Al-Masry Al-Youm* on August 17, 2017. The cartoon depicts a doctor standing next to a patient lying on a hospital bed. The doctor is holding on to what appears to be the empty pocket of the patient, examining the empty pocket, commenting, "You are suffering from a high inflation."

Several social scientists have discussed the porosity of the body to the environment in similar ways as captured by the notion of *ḍaghṭ*. Anthropologist Drew Leder, for example, argued that living organisms do not merely "gaze" upon the world, they literally "breathe" it in (Leder 1990:66). As stated previously, anthropologist Harris Solomon has, in similar ways, outlined the notion of "metabolic living" as a way to capture the intermingling of bodies, environments, and substances in relation to the onset and condition of diabetes (see Solomon 2016 for more on his work on diabetes in Mumbai). These arguments have increasingly been presented in different studies across different ethnographic settings, emphasizing the ways in which metabolism is not merely a physiological concept, but one that is closely linked to outward conditions as well (see, for example, Hardin 2015; Phillips et al. 2018; Sturtz Sreetharan et al. 2021; and Yates-Doerr 2019).

To the people that I worked with in Cairo who were diagnosed with type-2 diabetes, as well as to their relatives, the entanglements of bodies and environments were not theoretical, but literally experienced on a daily basis, captured through the notion of *ḍaghṭ* and the awareness of its connection to the onset and condition of, for example, type-2 diabetes. This placed the condition of diabetes, first, in the environment, then, in the body, causing people to reject the fundamental idea of type-2 diabetes as related to out-of-control individuals. The etiology of *ḍaghṭ* pointed, instead, to surroundings being out-of-control.

Anthropologist Sherine Hamdy has similarly argued from her work among kidney patients in Egypt that, "The connection that patients have made between their illnesses and failed state policies is not merely abstract or cerebral; it is a connection that they experience in material and bodily forms as well" (Hamdy 2012:183). In this same sense, Maha and others were not left bargaining prices at a local market place in the midst of Cairo, but also left bargaining against a global market and political attempts at stabilizing the economy and subsequent conditions set forth by the IMF; a global economy manifested in experiences of *ḍaghṭ* at a local market place in Cairo and subsequently in the bodies of Maha and others. To Maha and others, it was physically very evident how inflation rates specifically, and structural and political conditions more generally, potentially affected the onset and condition of type-2 diabetes.

#GotSugar? (October and November 2016)

Newspaper headlines, translated from Arabic when not originally published in English: "Supply Ministry introduces temporary solution to sugar shortage" (from *Al-Watan*, October 11, 2016); "Sweet-toothed Egypt endures a sugar crisis: 'People are going to snap'" (from *New York Times*, October 20, 2016); "Supply Ministry hunts monopolists, distributes sugar under police guard" (from *Al-Watan*, October 23, 2016); "Factories face potential halt in production amid sugar crisis" (from *Al-Shorouk*, October 25, 2016); "Courts issue expedited rulings to sentence 'sugar thieves' to prison" (from *Al-Shorouk*, October 26, 2016); "Supply Ministry sources: 134,000 tons of sugar to be imported within days" (from *Al-Watan*, October 27, 2016); "Egypt's sugar shortage a window on economic policy confusion" (from *Reuters*, November 2, 2016); "Minister of local development: Sugar crisis caused by rumors" (from *Al-Bawaba*, November 13, 2016); "Supply Ministry: 586 tons of sugar, oil and wheat arrive at Egyptian port" (from *Al-Ahram*, November 24, 2016).

Abundance and Scarcity

In the fall of 2016, while in Denmark on a break from my fieldwork, I received a notice from friends and acquaintances in Egypt that, suddenly, there was a shortage of sugar. The developing economic crisis had stirred concerns over spiking food prices in general, and sugar prices in particular. This had caused many Egyptians to buy an excess amount of sugar to store for later consumption when prices were expected to peak. In addition, suppliers withheld sugar upon realizing that they would be able to sell it at much higher prices in the near future. A combination of these factors, and a general increase of sugar prices on the global market, resulted in a sudden nationwide shortage of sugar.

The shortage incited much anger and uncertainty among many Egyptians, including many of the people that I knew well. At the time of the shortage one young male friend, for example, texted me, "What's next? There won't be any bread?" The anger among many Egyptians led Egyptian authorities to confiscate sugar for redistribution both from major factories who were using sugar in their production, as well as from people in the streets who were carrying more sugar than was deemed reasonable for personal use. Sugar was, reportedly, being sold on the black market at rates almost three times higher than the usual price of subsidized sugar – from approximately 5 Egyptian pounds per kilo to approximately 15 pounds per kilo (see, for example, Ashraf 2016; Hadid and Youssef 2016; Knecht and Dahan 2016; LMC 2017).

The resemblance in behavior and rhetoric in relation to this sweet white powder to that of drugs – the confiscation of drugs, holding of drugs, and illegal trading of drugs – is obvious. Jokes and satirical videos were as a result coming out of Egypt at the time of the shortage comparing the sugar addiction of the Egyptians to that of a drug addiction, ridiculing both the behavior of regular people and of the Egyptian authorities (see, for example, Abdelhadys 2016; Monks 2016). These included satirical hashtags such as the English #GotSugar?

The consumption of sugar (including high fructose corn syrup) is, in fact, relatively high in Egypt: Egyptians consume 36 kg of sugar per capita annually, which is a bit higher than the consumption in the United States and the EU. It compares to a global average of 23 kg per capita (LMC 2017:1–2). The importance of sugar to Egyptians is perhaps evident alone in the fact that it is subsidized by the state, as mentioned previously in this chapter (along with pasta, bread, rice, and cooking oil). It is used not only in tea, coffee, and juices, but also in more salty foods, such as couscous, soups, and sauces.

Quite a few of the people that I knew in Cairo at the time of the shortage actively participated in the spreading of jokes and videos about the sugar shortage on social media. Others found the shortage a very concerning matter, evident from angry online status updates or in text messages, such as the one cited above. In general, most people were concerned what other food items might suddenly be in short supply (Egypt, in fact, carries a long history of food riots on the grounds of shortages and increasing prices, see, for example, Mitchell 2002:249; Mittermaier 2014:62; Sutton et al. 2013:348–53 for accounts of such riots in the 1970s and later in 2007 and 2008). Other people that I knew well in Cairo felt directly affected by the fact that there was a shortage of sugar specifically. For example, one of Maha's distant relatives postponed her wedding due to the shortage and subsequent spikes in sugar prices. When I asked Maha about the matter, she responded with the following question, "How can they get married if they cannot even afford to serve their guests tea with sugar?" In other words, to some people in Cairo the sugar shortage had little effect, and was perhaps mostly a laughing matter, but to others it had a much greater impact. Even though Maha's relative did get married at a later point, in the words of Maha, the postponement had put a lot of "*ḍaghṭ*, pressure" on both the bride and groom and their families.

I emphasize the particular example of the sugar shortage here because the soothing effect of black tea with sugar was mentioned among almost everyone I worked with, as a way to relieve the body of experiences of *ḍaghṭ*. During the sugar shortage this was not an option, as few would drink their tea without sugar. This alone caused many of the people I knew in Cairo to frame the sugar shortage as causing "*ḍaghṭ kathīr*, a lot of pressure." In addition, the example illustrates the general concern with the overall supply of food and fluctuating prices of food which likewise were mentioned frequently by many of the people I knew in Cairo as causing them *ḍaghṭ kathīr*. To sum up in relation to the topic of food and calories, the onset of type-2 diabetes was not coupled with affluence or with an abundance of food by Maha, her mother, her in-laws and others. Rather, it was coupled with issues of deprivation and scarcity, and the experiences of *ḍaghṭ* brought on by such potential deprivation and scarcity. These experiences of *ḍaghṭ* were in turn brought on by a range of other issues, as evident throughout the above, related to the size, environment, and climate of Cairo; to economic and political uncertainties of prices, shortages, and potential riots; to conflicts within families over prices and priorities; and to the uncertainty of the quality of the food that one had to eat and serve to loved ones.

As stated previously in this chapter, international biomedical research does in fact relate type-2 diabetes to stress (see, for example, Corazon et al. 2010; Nielsen et al. 2008; and Tsiotra and Tsigos

2006), as well as to matters of historical periods of deprivation and scarcity. The latter risk factor is often referred to as the epigenetic risk factor of diabetes (see, for example, Zimmet 2017). Political scientist Timothy Mitchael has, in fact, outlined the outbreak of a simultaneous famine and malaria epidemic in parts of Upper Egypt at the time of the Second World War (Mitchell 2002:19–53). I could suggest here that this famine left future generations of Egyptians particularly vulnerable to type-2 diabetes, as has been discussed biomedically of famines elsewhere (Zimmet 2017). Three out of five of the families that I worked with in Cairo had, in fact, migrated from Upper Egypt one or two generations prior to the time of my fieldwork, and had thus potentially been exposed to this famine – and the epigenetic risk factor of such a famine. Metabolisms, in other words, are shaped not only in current bodies and environments (see, for example, Hardin 2015; Phillips et al. 2018; Sturtz Sreetharan et al. 2021; and Yates-Doerr 2019), but also in bodies and deprivations of past-time generations.

Eleven Suitors (May 2015)

It is late night, and Maha and I flip through the TV channels. We decide to watch an episode of a Egyptian soap opera called "*ʿAiza itgawiz*, I Want to Get Married." Each episode depicts the main female character trying to get engaged to a different man. Always in vain. We laugh our way through the episode. I turn to Maha and ask her about the time before she decided to marry Mustafa. Maha pulls her legs up under her dress and makes herself comfortable on the couch, as she starts reminiscing.

"One man came to my house, invited through my mother's friend. She never got married, so she made it her life's mission to get everyone else married." We laugh and Maha continues, "But that man was too old. Or he wasn't old but he looked old. He made me feel sick when I looked at him." Maha sticks her tongue out and makes a gagging sound. "She also sent another man to our house, but he was too short and childish-looking. After a while I would have looked like his mother." We both laugh again. Maha ponders for a while, and then continues, "Another man made less money than me, and in Egypt that doesn't work; a man goes insane if his wife makes more money than him, so he was no good. Another man moved to Dubai for work, and was really vague about whether or not he wanted to get married. Another man lived far away from my family and I wouldn't be able to walk home if we got into a fight. My father didn't like that; he died shortly thereafter, so I made sure to follow his advice." I nod and tell her that I understand. Maha continues after a while, "And then there were two other men, but they were both too shy. I laugh a lot and talk a lot so I can't marry a quiet and shy man," Maha says. I nod in agreement.

To my amazement, Maha continues down her list of suitors: "Two other men actually made a good impression. They were both nice and clever, but they had a bad reputation once we started asking around. One would tell everyone in his neighborhood about his personal problems and another one had a mother that loved drama." Maha sighs and shakes her head. "Oh, and one man didn't want me because I wanted to keep working after marriage." We sit in silence for a while. Amazed, I tell Maha that she had so many suitors. Maha smiles, "Yeah, but finally I agreed to marry Mustafa because he was the best of them all." I smile and ask Maha how it came about.

"Well, for years our families were talking about it. My mother told me that I wouldn't find someone better than Mustafa. Because he is my cousin, his family will always treat me well. And they have a lot of money. Or not a lot, but enough. And he is not bad looking ... But I kept refusing for years. I don't know. But then all the other men ... There was always something wrong with them and then finally Mustafa's sisters came to my house and told me that Mustafa really wanted to marry me. I told them no, but they told me to think about it before refusing it completely. After a couple of days, I agreed. And then we got engaged." I smile at Maha. "*Il-ḥamdū lillāh*, Thank God, it worked out," I say. "*Il-ḥamdū lillāh*," Maha responds as she smiles back at me.

Summary

I had known Maha for a couple of years before she married Mustafa, and had followed her efforts to get married closely. Throughout the process, Maha recounted the "*ḍaghṭ*, pressure" she felt to marry Mustafa in particular, and to find a suitable husband in general. Yet, the pressure did not stop with marriage. Already a couple of weeks into their marriage, Maha similarly talked about the "*ḍaghṭ*, pressure" put on her body to conceive a baby. Relatives and neighbors alike would stop her in the streets to ask if she was pregnant, all advised her to go to the doctor to learn if everything was "*maṣbūṭ*, right" with her body. Maha resisted their advice for a while, confiding in me that she did not believe anything was wrong with her body.

After six months of marriage, and still no pregnancy, she caved in to the pressure and decided to go to the doctor. The doctor assured her everything was fine, and demanded she go home, rest, and not listen to her neighbors. A month later, she was pregnant with her first child. Yet, the pregnancy added additional "*ḍaghṭ*, pressure" to Maha's body as environmental factors of, for example, moving around the market place, or enduring the hot climate in general, made her body swell and left her in a lot of pain. I draw on the example of Maha throughout the above to illustrate the ways in which people in Cairo – through their consistent exposure to the pressures of everyday life – believed that they might fall ill with type-2 diabetes at some point in their lives.

"Too much sugar in the blood, *sukkar kathīr fī il-dam*," had caused Maha's mother-in-law to fall ill with diabetes, according to Maha. The accumulated sugar, she explained, was brought on by the "*ḍaghṭ*, pressure" of having watched her neighbor burn to death. Ahmed, introduced in the previous chapter, similarly explained, "Pressure from life, *ḍaghṭ min il-ḥayā*, will result in pressure in your blood, *ḍaghṭ fī il-dam*." He added, "This is why you should drink tea. You can't drink tea when you are angry. You have to relax when you drink tea"; and thus the condition of type-2 diabetes was related momentarily to a shortage of sugar in the fall of 2016 that was preventing people with type-2 diabetes and others from enjoying the soothing and healing effects of sugary black tea. The reactions of Maha, Ahmed, and others to this specific sugar shortage illustrate the fact that they did not perceive "too much sugar in the blood" as related to the amount of sugars or other foods consumed per se. Rather, an accumulated sugar in the blood was brought on by experiences of *ḍaghṭ* which in turn were brought on by the omnipresent uncertainties in many different spheres of everyday life.

The people I worked with in Cairo who were diagnosed with type-2 diabetes and their relatives, in other words, did not relate the condition to neoliberal ideas of individual "lifestyle choices" or to notions of having enjoyed a life of abundance and affluence; rather, type-2 diabetes was related to a condition of deprivation and scarcity – of having enjoyed too little of what was considered good. In fact, when speaking of "the good life," people in Cairo commonly draw on the expression "*ḥayā ḥilwa*," which literally translates into "the sweet life." Fittingly, too little of what was considered "sweet," both literally and figuratively, was believed by Maha, Ahmed, and others to potentially cause the condition of type-2 diabetes. "*Maraḍ il-sukkar*," an illness of sugar, people in Cairo coined diabetes as an overall disease category. This seems a suitable summary of the above – although the relation of sugar and sweetness to type-2 diabetes was perceived somewhat differently than the one commonly outlined in biomedical literature, as well as by Egyptian healthcare personnel.

Note

1 Parts of this chapter have previously been published in *Culture, Medicine & Psychiatry* (Thorsen 2021).

References

Abdelhadys. 2016. Got Sugar? October 26, 2016. Cairo Scene. www.facebook.com/CairoScene/videos/1285726311458071/?pnref=story.

Ashraf, Nessma. 2016. Behind the Sugar Crisis. October 20, 2016. Al-Ahram Weekly. http://weekly.ahram.org.eg/News/17609.aspx.

Baer, Roberta, Susan Weller, Javier de Alba Garcia, and Ana Rocha. 2012. Ethnomedical and Biomedical Realities: Is There an Epidemiological Relationship between Stress-Related Folk Illnesses and Type 2 Diabetes? *Human Organization* 71(4): 339–347.

Barnard, Neal D., Susan M. Levin, Lise Gloede, and Rosendo Flores. 2018. Turning the Waiting Room into a Classroom: Weekly Classes Using a Vegan or a Portion-Controlled Eating Plan Improve Diabetes Control in a Randomized Translational Study. *Journal of the Academy of Nutrition and Dietetics* 118(6): 1072–1079.

Basyouny, Iman Farid. 1998. *Just a Gaze – Female Clientele of Diet Clinics in Cairo: An Ethnomedical Study*. The American University in Cairo Press.

Broom, Dorothy, and Andrea Whittaker. 2004. Controlling Diabetes, Controlling Diabetics: Moral Language in the Management of Diabetes Type 2. *Social Science & Medicine* 58(11): 2371–2382.

Charlton, Bruce G. 1992. Stress. *Journal of Medical Ethics* 18(3): 156–159.

Corazon, Sus Sola, Ulrika K. Stigsdotter, Anne Grete Claudi Jensen, and Kjell Nilsson. 2010. Development of the Nature-Based Therapy Concept for Patients with Stress-Related Illness at the Danish Healing Forest Garden Nacadia. *Journal of Therapeutic Horticulture* 20: 33–51.

Farag, Youssef M. K., and Mahmoud R. Gaballa. 2011. Diabesity: An Overview of a Rising Epidemic. *Nephrology Dialysis Transplantation* 26(1): 28–35.

Ferzacca, Steve. 2012. Diabetes and Culture. *Annual Review of Anthropology* 41: 411–426.

Flaherty, Michael G. 2011. *The Textures of Time: Agency and Temporal Experience*. Temple University Press.

Funahashi, Daena A. 2013. Wrapped in Plastic: Transformation and Alienation in the New Finnish Economy. *Cultural Anthropology* 28(1): 1–21.

Ghannam, Farha, and Hania Sholkamy. 2004. *Health and Identity in Egypt*. American University in Cairo Press.

Glasgow, Sara, and Ted Schrecker. 2016. The Double Burden of Neoliberalism? Noncommunicable Disease Policies and the Global Political Economy of Risk. *Health & Place* 39: 204–211.

Good, Byron J. 1977. The Heart of What's the Matter: The Semantics of Illness in Iran. *Culture, Medicine and Psychiatry* 1(1): 25–58.

Gray A., Threlkeld R.J. 2015. Nutritional Recommendations for Individuals with Diabetes. In: Endotext. MDText.com, Inc., South Dartmouth (MA); 2000.

Hadid, Diaa, and Nour Youssef. 2016. Sweet-Toothed Egypt Endures a Sugar Crisis: "People Are Going to Snap". October 20, 2016. The New York Times. www.nytimes.com/2016/10/21/world/middleeast/egypt-sugar-shortage.html.

Hamdy, Sherine F. 2008. When the State and Your Kidneys Fail: Political Etiologies in an Egyptian Dialysis Ward. *American Ethnologist* 35(4): 553–569.

Hamdy, Sherine F. 2012. *Our Bodies Belong to God: Organ Transplants, Islam, and the Struggle for Human Dignity in Egypt*. University of California Press.

Hardin, Jessica. 2015. Everyday Translation: Health Practitioners' Perspectives on Obesity and Metabolic Disorders in Samoa. *Critical Public Health* 25(2): 125–138.

Holodny, Elena. 2016. Egypt Just Massively Devalued Its Currency, and Here's What Happens Next. In *Business Insider*, November 3, 2016.

Ingold, T. 2000. *The Perception of the Environment: Essays on Livelihood, Dwelling and Skill*. Routledge.

Kalra, Sanjay, Jagat Jyoti Mukherjee, Subramanium Venkataraman, et al. 2013. Hypoglycemia: The Neglected Complication. *Indian Journal of Endocrinology and Metabolism* 17(5): 819.

Kleinman, Arthur. 1980. *Patients and Healers in the Context of Culture: An Exploration of the Borderland between Anthropology, Medicine, and Psychiatry*. University of California Press.

Knecht, Eric, and Maha el Dahan. 2016. Egypt's Sugar Shortage a Window on Economic Policy Confusion. Reuters, November 2. www.reuters.com/article/us-egypt-sugar/egypts-sugar-shortage-a-window-on-economic-policy-confusion-idUSKBN12X20O.

Kuriyama, Shigehisa. 1999. *The Expressiveness of the Body and the Divergence of Greek and Chinese Medicine*. Zone Books.

Leder, Drew. 1990. *The Absent Body*. University of Chicago Press.

Little, M., S. Humphries, K. Patel, and C. Dewey. 2017. Decoding the Type 2 Diabetes Epidemic in Rural India. *Medical Anthropology* 36(2): 96–110.

LMC. 2017. *Review of the Egyptian Sugar Sector*. medagri.org.

Long, A. E., T. E. Prewitt, J. S. Kaufman, et al. 1998. Weight-Height Relationships among Eight Populations of West African Origin: The

Case against Constant BMI Standards. *International Journal of Obesity* 22: 842–846.

Lupton, Deborah. 2013. *Fat*. Routledge.

Mitchell, Timothy. 2002. *Rule of Experts: Egypt, Techno-Politics, Modernity*. University of California Press.

Mittermaier, Amira. 2014. Bread, Freedom, Social Justice: The Egyptian Uprising and a Sufi Khidma. *Cultural Anthropology* 29(1): 54–79.

Mol, Annemarie. 2008a. *The Logic of Care: Health and the Problem of Patient Choice*. Routledge.

Mol, Annemarie. 2008b. I Eat an Apple: On Theorizing Subjectivities. *Subjectivity* 22(1): 28–37.

Monks, Kieron. 2016. Sugar Crash Sparks Crisis in Egypt. CNN, November 2. https://edition.cnn.com/2016/11/02/africa/egypt-sugar-crash/index.html.

Nielsen, Naja Rod, Tage S. Kristensen, Peter Schnohr, and Morten Grønbæk. 2008. Perceived Stress and Cause-Specific Mortality among Men and Women: Results from a Prospective Cohort Study. *American Journal of Epidemiology* 168(5): 481–491.

Phillips, Tarryn, Celia McMichael, and Michael O'Keefe. 2018. "We Invited the Disease to Come to Us": Neoliberal Public Health Discourse and Local Understanding of Non-Communicable Disease Causation in Fiji. *Critical Public Health* 28(5): 560–572.

Qureshi, Kaveri. 2013. Body Politics among Middle-Aged Migrant Pakistani Women. *The Journal of the Royal Anthropological Institute* 19(1): 120–137.

Reubi, David, Clare Herrick, and Tim Brown. 2016. The Politics of Non-Communicable Diseases in the Global South. *Health & Place* 39: 179–187.

Rock, Melanie. 2003. Sweet Blood and Social Suffering: Rethinking Cause-Effect Relationships in Diabetes, Distress, and Duress. *Medical Anthropology* 22(2): 131–174.

Schoenberg, Nancy E., Elaine M. Drew, Eleanor P. Stoller, and Cary S. Kart. 2005. Situating Stress: Lessons from Lay Discourses on Diabetes. *Medical Anthropology Quarterly* 19(2): 171–193.

Seligman, Rebecca, Emily Mendenhall, Maria D. Valdovinos, Alicia Fernandez, and Elizabeth A. Jacobs. 2015. Self-Care and Subjectivity among Mexican Diabetes Patients in the United States. *Medical Anthropology Quarterly* 29(1): 61–79.

Selye, Hans. 1976. Forty Years of Stress Research: Principal Remaining Problems and Misconceptions. *Canadian Medical Association Journal* 115(1): 53–56.

Sheikh, Bassem Y. 2016. The Role of Prophetic Medicine in the Management of Diabetes Mellitus: A Review of Literature. *Journal of Taibah University Medical Science* 11(4): 339–352.

Solomon, Harris. 2016. *Metabolic Living: Food, Fat, and the Absorption of Illness in India*. Duke University Press.

Sturtz Sreetharan, Cindi, Alexandra Brewis, Jessica A. Hardin, Sarah Trainer, and Amber Wutich. 2021. *Fat in Four Cultures: A Global Ethnography of Weight*. University of Toronto Press.

Sutton, David, Nefissa Naguib, Leonidas Vournelis, and Maggie Dickinson. 2013. Food and Contemporary Protest Movements. *Food, Culture & Society* 16(3): 345–366.

Tabishat, Mohammed. 2000. Al-Daght: Pressures of Modern Life in Cairo. *In Situating Globalization: Views from Egypt*. C. Nelson, and S. Rouse, eds. Pp. 203–230. Transcript.

Thorsen, Mille Kjærgaard. 2021. Under Pressure: Living with Diabetes in Cairo. *Culture, Medicine and Psychiatry*.

Trnka, Susanna, and Catherine Trundle. 2017. *Competing Responsibilities: The Politics and Ethics of Contemporary Life*. Susanna Trnka, and Catherine Trundle, eds. Duke University Press.

Tsiotra, Panayoula C., and Constantine Tsigos. 2006. Stress, the Endoplasmic Reticulum, and Insulin Resistance. *Annals of the New York Academy of Sciences* 1083(1): 63–76.

Weaver, Lesley Jo. 2018. *Sugar and Tension: Diabetes and Gender in Modern India*. Rutgers University Press.

WHO. 2016. *Global Report on Diabetes*. World Health Organization

Williams, Gareth. 2002. Chronic Illness and the Pursuit of Virtue in Everyday Life. *In Worlds of Illness: Biographical and Cultural Perspectives on Health and Disease*. A. Radley, ed. Routledge, 104–120.

Yates-Doerr, Emily. 2019. *The Weight of Obesity*. University of California Press.

Young, Allan. 1980. The Discourse on Stress and the Reproduction of Conventional Knowledge. *Social Science & Medicine* 14(3): 133–146.

Zimmet, Paul Z. 2017. Diabetes and Its Drivers: The Largest Epidemic in Human History? *Clinical Diabetes and Endocrinology* 3(1): 1–8.

4 Drugs

In the previous chapters, I have examined the ways in which "diabesity" is foregrounded as the most essential etiology of type-2 diabetes within international medical research and guidelines, as well as among healthcare personnel in Egypt; and how this specific etiology clashes with an etiology linking experiences of *ḍaghṭ* to the onset and condition of type-2 diabetes among those I worked with in Cairo who were diagnosed with the condition and their relatives. In this chapter, I turn to elaborate on the overall question of *why* "diabesity" is emphasized within international medical research and guidelines over other etiologies also acknowledged within biomedical research. I pick up on some of the arguments presented in the previous chapter of the ways in which "fatness" historically in Europe and North America has been linked to matters of "deviant and uncontrolled physical practices" (Lupton 2013:49–51).

Anthropological literature also referenced in the previous chapter (see, for example, Glasgow and Schrecker 2016; Phillips, McMichael, and O'Keefe 2018; Reubi, Herrick, and Brown 2016; and Trnka and Trundle 2017) has critically examined how such understandings have placed the moral responsibility of type-2 diabetes primarily within the realm of the individual, its solution theoretically simple: to lose and to control one's weight. In this chapter, I will elaborate on these arguments in relation to my research in Cairo by examining the ways in which such neoliberal understandings of health affect also the promotion of specific drugs used to treat type-2 diabetes globally, including among people in Cairo.

Much has been written anthropologically on the topic of pharmaceuticals and the pharmaceutical industry more generally (evident, for example, in the following literature reviews on the topic: Geest, Hardon, and Whyte 1996; Hardon and Sanabria 2017). A majority of these studies focus on the relation between clinical trials, investors, and governments, exploring the dilemma of promoting health

DOI: 10.4324/9781003327684-4

and curing illness coupled with a pharmaceutical industry whose main motivation is to maximize profits through maintaining long-time drug consumers (see, for example, Dumit 2012; Rajan 2017; Sismondo 2015). Other studies have focused on the consumption of pharmaceuticals, outlining how drugs are actualized when they are prescribed and used, dissolved, and absorbed in individual bodies and environments (see, for example, Landecker 2016; Nading 2017; Wilson 2015). Anthropologists Anita Hardon and Emilia Sanabria, for example, argue that there are no pure pharmaceutical objects: "Matter is always in movement, being molded and transformed by human and nonhuman processes and practices" (Hardon and Sanabria 2017:118–19).

In this chapter, I draw on the above bodies of work to discuss the ways in which neoliberal ideas of health and etiologies, and the pharmaceutical industry and its medicalization of individual bodies, mutually affect and enhance each other. I argue that a tendency of solutions to precede and define social problems (Spector and Kitsuse 2001) is evident in the ways available medical solutions targeting individual bodies contribute to defining the "problem" of type-2 diabetes as primarily one of the individual. While political and structural conditions cannot be medicated, individual bodies exposed to such conditions can.

I first focus on the use of metformin, sold in Egypt under the brand name Glucophage; a blood sugar lowering drug most commonly used in Egypt to treat type-2 diabetes. I show how the intended effect of metformin, for example, to induce a weight loss (among other effects), caused people in Cairo to question this drug as a suitable treatment. I argue that the reluctance to take metformin among some of the people I worked with in Cairo stemmed in part from an overall resistance to accept the etiology of "diabesity," as portrayed in the previous chapter, and thus of obesity as a legitimate target of type-2 diabetes treatment.

In the second part of the chapter, I move from an empirical focus on the use of metformin specifically to a more general focus on pharmaceuticals, arguing that an awareness among people in Cairo of drugs as matter always in movement, to paraphrase Hardon and Sanabria (Hardon and Sanabria 2017:118–19), manifested in great uncertainties among the people I worked with and met in passing. These uncertainties frequently resulted in adjustments and disruptions of treatment with pharmaceutical drugs among people in Cairo – without the consulting of doctors or other healthcare personnel. The uncertainties did not relate solely to the theoretical workings of drugs (and their specific targeting in the body, for example, to induce weight loss as outlined in the above case of metformin), but also to more general concerns, for example, of the potential contamination of drugs or geopolitics of drugs. Similar to the arguments presented in the previous chapter on food, the circumstance that pharmaceutical drugs had traveled through many different environments – biological, but also social and political environments – and thus had potentially been affected by a wide range of factors before finally reaching the hands of the consumer was a known and well-debated fact among people in Cairo. But this known fact in turn cemented a host of unknowns, causing great uncertainty as to which drugs were safe to take and which were not. In other words, people in Cairo were very aware that the pharmaceutical industry – manifested in drugs sold to medicate bodies and ailments – was not a neutral industry, but an industry with specific, yet often uncertain, agendas and motives.

Overall, this chapter discusses the ways in which the pharmaceutical industry enhances a neoliberal understanding of type-2 diabetes in its attempts to medicate individual bodies and their so-called obesity; however, the chapter simultaneously discusses the ways in which people in Cairo were reluctant to merely accept this idea – acutely aware of the ways in which type-2 diabetes in their perspective was rather related to experiences of *ḍaghṭ* caused by a great many uncertainties in many spheres of everyday life, including those related, for example, to the supply and use of pharmaceutical drugs.

Taher's Mother Asks an Important Question (October 2015)

It's Friday night and Taher and I walk under a highway bridge in downtown Cairo. It's dark and the streets are getting busy with families traveling back and forth to visit other family members. Taher recalls his morning shift as a medical intern in the emergency room at one of the university hospitals in Cairo. A Syrian woman had given birth to her son in the middle of the emergency room, and the staff were so few and so busy that no one had been there to assist the woman. Her baby had dropped directly on the floor.

Another woman had collapsed outside of the gates of the hospital with a document from another hospital stating that she was diagnosed with meningitis. Initially, none of the staff had dared to touch her, afraid they might catch meningitis themselves. Taher and another young colleague eventually stepped in to help her.

"You know, we barely have a pair of gloves we can use when treating patients like her," Taher adds, explaining why so few of the staff were willing to help the woman. I try to contemplate all of the stories as we go, listening intensely in silence.

"And then we had a lot of broken limbs," Taher finally concludes. "It was a crazy day … oh, and one woman came to the ER because her blood sugar was really, really high. She refused to take her diabetes medication saying 'the doctor said the pills will help me lose weight, but I am not fat.' She was really fat," Taher laughs. "And kind of stupid," he adds.

Finally, we reach the gates of Taher's aunt's house, in the heart of Shubra. The house is packed with people of all ages. Children are running, laughing, yelling, eating popcorn, playing with balloons and their cell phones. Everyone is talking, eating, drinking soda, lemonade, tea, and coffee. Taher leaves me with his mother, aunts, and female cousins. "I'll be right back," he says. Someone asks me if I want tea. I nod and smile. The women are discussing someone's husband who apparently wants to take a second wife.

"I would be so angry if that was my husband!" one of Taher's female cousins says. "I would leave him!" another one declares.

One of the cousins changes the topic and asks another cousin which vitamins she should take while pregnant. They discuss the recommendations given by their different doctors. Another cousin chimes in. Someone interrupts the girls, and asks if they heard that one of their neighbors is really sick. "Something with the heart," she adds. They talk back and forth, attempting to clarify what exactly the neighbor is suffering from. I don't catch the name of the condition, but finally one of the older aunts declares indifferently, "*Da ʿādī*, that's normal." A cousin hands me a cup of tea. I thank her and take a sip, trying to keep up with the conversation.

One of Taher's aunts asks his mother what she takes for her diabetes.

"Glucophage," she says. "Once a day," she raises a finger.

"A small, white pill?" the aunt asks.

"Yes," Taher's mother confirms.

"I heard it is really bad for your kidneys," the aunt says, leaning closer to Taher's mother. "My son-in-law told me," she adds, "he looked it up on the internet." Taher's mother doesn't respond. "It also makes you lose weight," the aunt elaborates. "It's not good for you," she finally declares, shaking her head. The aunt explains to Taher's mother that her doctor told her to take "Glucophage." "But I am not going to," she firmly states. "It's not good for you," she repeats once again.

"But it's only a small pill and only once a day ..." Taher's mother finally responds. The aunt shakes her head again.

Taher enters the living room. He is chasing one of the small children with a toy sword. His mother calls him out. "Taher ... *ya Taher ... ta'āla henna*, come over here." Taher tickles the child, and walks across the room.

"What?" he asks, looking at his mother.

"Your aunt tells me the pill you give me is not good for me," his mother says.

"Well, that's not true," Taher sighs. "You have diabetes, you need to take the pill," he declares.

"But it's bad for my kidneys, and I might lose weight," Taher's mother argues.

"The pill makes your blood sugar *maṣbūṭ*, precise, and yes, you might lose weight, but that will only benefit you even more," Taher explains patiently.

"How?" Taher's aunt asks sharply, eyes zooming in on Taher. Taher looks back at her.

"Well ... it will help her blood sugar even more," he says.

"But you already said it's *maṣbūṭ*, precise," the aunt responds.

"Because she takes the pill!" Taher says. The women all laugh.

Taher turns to his mother. "Look *ya mama*, please just take the pill. I know what I am talking about, I would not give you the pill if I thought it was dangerous." Taher looks at his mother for a while.

"Okay okay," his mother finally says, patting his cheek. Taher gives her a blank stare, toy sword still in his hand.

"I check your blood sugar every week, I will know if you stop taking the pill," he says. All the women laugh again.

"But I am not even really fat ..." Taher's mother says.

"Well ..." Taher says, shrugging his shoulders, quickly making a run for it out of the living room.

Treating Diabesity Medically (Introducing Taher)

I first met Taher during my fieldwork in Cairo in 2015, when he was finishing his last internship at one of the university hospitals in Cairo. At the time, Taher was in his late 20s and very driven by his work. In addition to his internship at the university hospital, he was working shifts at a private hospital on the outskirts of Cairo, and volunteering as a medical aid at an organization assisting refugees. Taher was an only child. His parents had recently divorced when I first met him, but they were still living close to each other in the downtown neighborhood of Shubra. Taher lived mostly with his mother. His father was a pharmacist, and owned his own pharmacy. Taher's mother had been assisting in the pharmacy throughout Taher's upbringing, but was now retired and living primarily off her late father's pension, along with Taher's contributions to the household. Taher's mother (and aunt) had both been diagnosed with type-2 diabetes several years before my first fieldwork stay in Cairo. In short, the family provided me with great insights into the topic of type-2 diabetes – both from the perspective of a young doctor, from that of an experienced pharmacist, and from that of Taher's mother and aunt.

In Egypt, employees in the public sector, as well as students at public universities and schools, are covered by the public Health Insurance Organisation (HIO). In theory, the insurance provides medical services, including medicine, free of charge or for only a small fee. Approximately 55% of the Egyptian population is insured under the HIO (Wanis 2015:60). Those belonging to the wealthier segments of Egyptian society usually have some kind of private insurance in relation to their jobs. Others pay out-of-pocket or may apply for coverage from the Egyptian state on a case-by-case basis. In the case of diabetes medicine, everyone within the families that I worked with paid for their own medicine out-of-pocket, whether covered by the public health insurance or not. As to the reason for this, they all pointed to the hassle of working through the bureaucratic process to retrieve the free medicine from the public healthcare system, as compared to the relatively low price of the most commonly used diabetes medication. Prior to the economic crisis that hit in 2016, Egypt had some of the lowest prices of medicine in the region of the Middle East and North Africa. This was partially due to a strict regulation of prices (in negotiation with pharmaceutical companies and other key players) and due to state subsidies on certain pharmaceutical categories, including insulin (Wanis 2015:75).

Metformin is one of the cheapest diabetes drugs available on the Egyptian market. In Egypt, it is known most commonly under the brand name of Glucophage. It works primarily by reducing the amount of sugar produced in the liver, and thus the amount of sugar released into the bloodstream. In addition, it improves the effect of insulin on the body. It is also known to suppress the appetite, and thus to potentially induce a weight loss (Heine et al. 2006; Nye and Herrington 2011). Toward the end of 2018, one package of 50 tablets of 500mg metformin was sold for approximately 15 Egyptian pounds (gone up from about 10 Egyptian pounds at the beginning of my fieldwork in 2015 prior to the economic crisis of

2016).[1] Those advised by their doctors in Cairo to take metformin were recommended to take up to 2000mg a day (1–4 tablets). In other words, a package of 50 500mg tablets would commonly last from 12 to 50 days.

Most of those within the families that I worked with in Cairo who were diagnosed with type-2 diabetes had been advised by their doctors to take metformin, and most did as prescribed. However, some of them, such as Taher's mother and aunt, as well as other patients that I encountered during medical consultations across various clinics in Cairo, were reluctant to merely accept the workings of this specific drug – particularly its potential to induce a weight loss. In their perspective, metformin appeared a medical manifestation of the etiology of "diabesity." As obesity in their understanding was linked to neither the onset nor the condition of type-2 diabetes, weight loss was not considered a desirable effect of a diabetes drug.

Anthropologists Joseph Dumit and Linda Hunt have argued that national and international guidelines of diagnostic criteria, as well as globally recommended treatment guidelines, define type-2 diabetes as a condition in need of specific treatment. Dumit specifically outlines how diagnostic criteria for different types of diabetes have changed over time, as different diabetes medications have become available on the global market. This includes the establishment of a newfound category of "prediabetes," forming also a new group of people in sudden need of medical attention (Dumit 2012:114–15). He argues that, "Diabetes is regularly invoked as a paradigmatic template for many conditions that were previously not thought of as illnesses" (Dumit 2012:7). In similar ways as Dumit, Hunt argues that the pharmaceutical industry and its affiliates "have fabricated a diabetes 'epidemic' and treatment standards that require heavy use of pharmaceuticals" (Hunt 2017:1). Dumit and Hunt both outline how the primary ambition of the pharmaceutical industry is to pursue profits for their shareholders, not to cure illnesses as such. Hunt argues, "This they accomplish [...] by creating and sustaining markets" (Hunt 2017:1). "A life on drugs," Dumit sums up in the title of his book (Dumit 2012). In other words, both Dumit and Hunt argue that medical solutions made available by the pharmaceutical industry often define, and redefine, the problem or condition of chronic illnesses such as type-2 diabetes.

Sociologists Malcolm Spector and John Kitsuse first discussed the relation between "problems" and "solutions" in the 1980s, arguing that solutions tend to precede problems. More specifically, they argued that responses and solutions by institutional agencies define conditions as troublesome in specific ways. Thus, problems do not precede solutions; rather, solutions precede problems. Spector and Kitsuse elaborated that "solutions produce problems by providing the framework within which those problems can be stated [...] Every experience of displeasure and dissatisfaction has its origin in the availability, if not promise, of remedies, cures, reforms, and solutions for such troubles" (Spector and Kitsuse 2001:84). Anthropologists Steffen Jöhncke, Mette Svendsen, and Susan Whyte have elaborated on these arguments pointing to the ways in which "solutions" produce certain bearers of a "problem"; bearers of certain attributes that make them suited for the solution (Jöhncke, Svendsen, and Whyte 2004:392).

Drawing on the above overall arguments, I argue that the same mechanisms were evident in Cairo. Available treatment solutions to type-2 diabetes (such as metformin and other drugs working in part by inducing a weight loss, but also other treatment solutions such as specific dietary advice, recommendations to stay physically active, monitor calories, and the like) contributed to a foregrounding of a specific "problem" of type-2 diabetes and thus of specific attributes of the "bearers" of this problem. The "solution" of weight loss defined type-2 diabetes as a "problem" of obesity – in turn characterizing the bearers of type-2 diabetes as per definition obese.

I want here to extend the critical discussions of a neoliberal emplacement of the moral responsibility of type-2 diabetes primarily within the realm of the individual to emphasize also the ways in which the pharmaceutical industry contributes to or enhances this individualization of health. Such a focus, I argue, excludes political and other structural conditions from being included as part of the problem of type-2 diabetes. In other words, available solutions to type-2 diabetes promoted by a pharmaceutical industry that solely and powerfully medicates individual bodies undermines political and other structural inequities of type-2 diabetes of which a solution is not so easily available, however equally necessary. This became very evident in Cairo as those diagnosed with type-2 diabetes had come to resist, for example, political and medical uncertainties by maintaining an atmosphere of uncertainty themselves; persistently questioning the motives of, for example, doctors, but also of pharmaceuticals and medical companies in general.

Regarding metformin, this was also evident in the ways quite a few raised concerns as to whether or not metformin would damage their kidneys, despite their doctors reassuring them that it would not. Biomedically, metformin is not believed to damage the kidneys as such, but to pose a danger to already impaired kidneys.

Metformin thus carries a warning label not to be used by patients with impaired kidneys (a common late complication among people with diabetes) due to the risk of developing the potentially fatal condition of lactic acidosis (see, for example, Inzucchi et al. 2014; Nye and Herrington 2011). Considering the fact that people diagnosed with type-2 diabetes are at high risk of developing impaired kidneys, and that few of the people I came across in Cairo who were diagnosed with the condition had their kidneys medically assessed on a regular basis, the likelihood that someone was suffering from an undiagnosed impairment of the kidneys was relatively high.

Regardless, Taher and other doctors that I knew in Cairo regularly addressed the issue with their patients, maintaining that metformin did not damage the kidneys as such. One doctor told me specifically during an interview, "Yes, patients raise this question [of the relation between metformin and kidney damage] all the time, because the warning is right there on the box! Only, they misunderstand the warning, and believe the drug to be generally unsafe."

Let me be clear: I am not diminishing the need for medical treatment of type-2 diabetes as such. However, I do wish to challenge the ways in which the pharmaceutical industry – underpinned by international medical research and guidelines – contributes to undermining other known risk factors of type-2 diabetes (and other ailments for that matter) because they cannot be medicated. In other words, international medical research and guidelines allow the pharmaceutical industry to dominate etiologies and treatments of a condition far more complex than merely related to obesity and to a matter of individual health and behavior alone.

By the time of my second fieldwork stay in Cairo in 2017, Taher had graduated from medical school and was now working in a public clinic as a general practitioner. The clinic was situated in a mosque in downtown Cairo. According to Taher, the mosque had donated its space to the government for it to run a public clinic in the neighborhood. Having graduated from a public university, Taher had to work in the clinic before being able to apply for a specialty. In the following empirical encounter from Taher's workplace, I turn to focus more generally on the topic of pharmaceuticals, and how the consumption of pharmaceuticals in general was connected with great uncertainties among people in Cairo.

The General Practitioner's Office (March 2017)

We are in downtown Cairo, close to the Abdeen Palace. We come around a corner and face the mosque in which Taher now works as a general practitioner. We pass a woman sitting next to a big pile of garlic. She eyes us as we go by. Two young women have set up a table in front of the mosque, with flyers spread out across the table and freezer containers placed by their feet. Taher whispers in English, "It's a polio vaccination campaign. Polio was eradicated in Egypt, but it's back now ..."

Taher and I enter the mosque, and we climb the stairway to the clinic on the second floor. Taher signs his name in a book; "I have to register," he whispers in English. I follow Taher into one of the consultation rooms, and we both greet the nurse inside. She wears a uniform of dark blue pants, a white shirt, white scarf, and clogs. Taher is wearing his own casual clothes; jeans, sneakers, and a t-shirt. Taher finds his seat behind the doctor's desk and tells me to take the seat next to him. The desk is lopsided, paint is coming off where Taher and other doctors have rested their arms and pulled out the drawers. I notice that one of the drawers does not close properly, and there are medical brochures and pills inside the drawer.

The walls of the consultation room are plastered with posters displaying various messages in a mix of English and Arabic. Some posters look professional and printed by medical companies and the WHO, while others look homemade. One such sign reads in English, "Clean hands save lives." It is printed on a piece of paper stuffed inside of a dirty plastic sleeve. Taher grabs a stethoscope, a pen, and a bottle of water out of his bag. He leaves it all out on the desk. The nurse calls the name of the first patient, and there is a steady stream of patients from this point forward. During the first two hours, 30 patients consult Taher with a variety of medical issues, mainly the flu, pneumonia, gout, throat infections, and undefined pain or discomfort. One teenage girl complains that her heart is beating at an uneven rate. A couple of other patients complain that their blood pressure is too high. One little girl appears to suffer from asthma. Others appear to suffer from diabetes and dysregulated blood sugar. Taher hands out aspirin, antibiotics, and antihypertensive medication from the drawer. Other patients are given sticky notes with names of drugs to buy from the pharmacy, or lab work that needs to be done. Others are told to go to a different doctor or a different clinic altogether.

A young woman enters the consultation room with her mother, and Taher tells the nurse to close the door behind them. The woman is very pale, and moves slowly across the room. She sits down opposite Taher and immediately explains that the clinic gave her some medicine a couple of days ago, but the medicine is making her feel really sick. She explains that she was told to inject the medicine once in the morning and once at night for an entire week, but she refuses to keep going.

"I have only been taking the medicine for a day, and my whole body is aching," she says. "I can barely stand on my feet," she adds. Taher asks about the medicine. The woman hands Taher an ampule and then another. He examines them briefly.

"Why were you supposed to take these?" he asks.

The woman explains that she has had diarrhea and a fever for more than a week. "I think that's why," she says. Taher explains that one ampule contains antibiotics and the other B-vitamins.

"You should really keep taking these once you have started," Taher says. "You feel sick from your diarrhea, not from the medicine," he adds.

The young woman quietly mumbles, "Okay."

The young woman's mother takes her daughter's seat opposite Taher. She starts explaining that she has both hepatitis C and diabetes, and that her joints are aching badly.

"I am in so much pain," she elaborates. "I cannot even open a bottle of water, my wrists hurt that badly," she says, pointing toward Taher's water bottle. Taher asks what medicine she is taking. "Nothing. I did take a pill for my diabetes, but I stopped. Someone told me the pill was bad for my kidneys." Taher sighs quietly.

"No, diabetes is bad for your kidneys, the pill will help you," he says.

Noise is coming from the busy waiting room. Taher glances toward the door, and then tells the woman, "Look … I have a lot of people waiting. It is better if you see another doctor, someone who knows a lot about diabetes. Do you know one?" The woman nods. "It's better," Taher says again, as he opens the drawer and hands the woman some aspirin. "For the pain," he says. The woman shakes her head.

"I have plenty at home," she says. Taher drops the pills back into the drawer. The woman then suggests that maybe her blood pressure is too high. Taher quickly measures her blood pressure.

"It's fine," he observes.

A young woman suddenly enters the room without knocking, interrupting the consultation. She promptly throws what looks to be lab results on the desk in front of Taher.

"Do they look normal to you?" she asks while looking intensely at Taher. Without uttering a word, Taher quickly scans the paper. I can tell that the blood sugar levels stated on the lab results are extremely high. Taher stamps the paper and signs it, and then tells the woman to go back to the lab for another round of measurements.

"No, these are not right," he says. "If these were accurate, you would be in a coma or dead by now." The young woman snatches the paper.

"That's what I thought," she says as she turns to leave.

The Uncertainties of Drugs

Rather than merely trust in the supposed positive effects of drugs – and in the reassurances given, for example, by doctors and pharmaceutical companies – the people that I worked with in Cairo frequently questioned not only the workings of specific drugs, but also for example, the potential contamination of drugs, as well as the potential hidden agendas of pharmaceutical companies. Anthropologists Adriana Petryna and Arthur Kleinman have outlined how trust in the workings of pharmaceutical drugs is gained by medical companies and governments through the use of rhetoric and "expert know-how," "surveillance guidelines," "trustworthy standards" and the like (Petryna and Kleinman 2006:10–12). In Cairo, I argue, such rhetoric and promises did little to reassure people of the workings and safety of pharmaceuticals. Rather, as was the case of medical advice in general or attempts by authorities to control the narrative of political events, it did quite the contrary; it maintained a persistent questioning of the pharmaceutical industry and its products.

Uncertainties in relation to the use of pharmaceutical drugs were facilitated first and foremost by stories circulating among relatives, friends, colleagues, and strangers, online as well as in newspapers and on other media platforms. These stories revolved around the potential side effects of certain drugs, as evident in the previous empirical encounters regarding concerns about the relation between metformin and kidney damage. Other examples that were talked about in the families that I was working with revolved, for example, around the specific use of Sovaldi, a drug used to treat hepatitis C. This drug was widely believed among members of the families that I was working with to cause liver cancer (however, all of the doctors I spoke to in Egypt linked hepatitis C to the possible onset of liver cancer, not Sovaldi). Other concerns expressed across the families revolved around the potential risks of blood clots and certain types of cancer in relation to the use of certain birth control (both biomedically acknowledged as a risk of many types of hormonal birth control). This point was emphasized particularly in

Maha's family, as her sister-in-law had previously been hospitalized with a blood clot in her leg. This had been linked by doctors in the hospital to the use of a certain type of birth control (prescribed by a different doctor originally).

In addition to concerns over side effects of certain drugs, other concerns revolved around the use of counterfeit medicine, expired medicine, or medicine that had gone bad from human neglect, for example, from not being stored at the right temperatures or from not being released from the Egyptian customs before turning bad (however, subsequently sold through local pharmacies). One specific example from the time of my fieldwork in Cairo in the summer of 2015 illustrates some of these concerns rather well. For example, a story suddenly surfaced (in the media, as well as across the families that I was working with at the time, including Maha's family) that 27 infants had been poisoned from an intravenous rehydration solution administered to treat dehydration at public hospitals across the governorate of Beni Suef. Ultimately, four children died. The Egyptian Ministry of Health named a Cairene drug company as the manufacturer of the solution, but the company itself declined ever having manufactured such a drug (El-Fekki 2015). Uncertainties in relation to the origin of drugs were commonly evoked on the grounds of similar stories.

In addition to the above, sudden fluctuations on the pharmaceutical market in relation to the availability and prices of certain medicines cemented the geopolitical contexts in which pharmaceutical drugs are produced and sold. This was evident, for example, as rumors circulated toward the end of 2017 about the potential consequences of a boycott of American products, including certain medicines. The boycott was a response to President Donald Trump's decision to move the American Embassy in Israel to Jerusalem. Specifically, stories were circulating that such a boycott would harm Egyptian patients, causing a shortage of a range of pharmaceutical drugs. A penicillin shortage did, in fact, affect the Egyptian drug market in late 2017, but it was eventually linked to a high-ranking Egyptian official, not to President Donald Trump. Apparently, the official had attempted to manipulate the penicillin market by moving the import of penicillin from a state-owned company to his own private company, creating a void in the market as opposed to a monopoly (Tawfeek 2017). In general, the economic crisis from 2016 and onwards caused prices of pharmaceutical drugs in Egypt to increase greatly (initially by 25%, eventually by 50% of the original price), affecting not only consumers, but also the ability of the pharmacists to stock up on medicine. This caused a range of shortages, including a shortage of certain diabetes drugs. There were stories in the media particularly about the unwillingness of medical companies to lower their prices to support Egyptian consumers.

Many of the concerns outlined above were visible in headlines from Egyptian newspapers throughout the years of my research. Examples of such headlines include (translated here from Arabic into English): "Confusion follows new price increases in pharmaceuticals market" (from *Al-Wafd*, May 19, 2016); "Pharmacists Syndicate: Counterfeit medications flooding market are killing patients" (from *Al-Watan*, August 16, 2016); "Chemotherapy treatment for children stops due to lack of medication" (from *Al-Dostour*, October 23,2016); "Pharmaceuticals for kidney, liver, diabetes and heart patients disappear from market, as Health Minister's meeting with pharmacists fails" (from *Al-Dostour*, November 16, 2016); "Crisis between pharmaceutical companies and Health Ministry escalates: 146 medications disappear" (from *Al-Wafd*, November 21, 2016); "Secret behind smuggled pharmaceuticals: Illegal operations generate US$10 bn at 500% profit" (from Al-*Wafd*, January 5, 2017); "Pharmacists Union: 1236 drugs missing from markets. Health Ministry: Inaccurate information" (from *Al-Masry Al-Youm*, April 17, 2017); "Ministry of Health warns of counterfeit medicine" (from *Al-Wafd*, July 19,2017); "Head of Pharmacists Syndicate: Hepatitis C medicine available at hospitals 'totally safe'" (from *Al-Masry Al-Youm*, August 9, 2017); "The 'Penicillin crisis' continues: Hospitals unable to help as patients in need of medicine line up in front of pharmacies" (from *Al-Gomhurriya*, December 11, 2017); "Health Ministry warning: 7 cancer and eye drop drugs in market are counterfeit" (from *Al-Watan*, May 21, 2018); "Pharmacies defy Health Ministry warning, sell carcinogenic drugs [drugs believed to cause cancer]" (from *Al-Watan*, August 10, 2018).

The close interactions of the pharmaceutical market with, for example, geopolitical and economic issues added to a sentiment of uncertainty in relation to the origin of drugs, authenticity of drugs, and steady availability of drugs, making the potential effects of the various environments through which pharmaceutical drugs travel before finally reaching the consumer the more visible. Anthropologists Geest, Hardon, and Whyte draw on the analytical notion of a "life cycle" of pharmaceuticals to capture this process. They argue, "As commodities, pharmaceuticals have lives and 'deaths' far more significant than their shelf lives and expiration dates" (Geest, Hardon, and Whyte 1996:171). Put differently, pharmaceuticals pass through many spheres of social life. They are, for example, produced by private or public entities in specific geopolitical, socioeconomic, and historical contexts; they must undergo tests to be released to a broader market; must travel across borders and local customs to reach local consumers; they are prescribed in various ways by doctors and other healthcare providers; and are finally consumed in equally many different ways by different people. Geest, Hardon, and Whyte sum up, "Each life stage is characterized by a specific context and particular actors" (Geest, Hardon, and Whyte 1996:156). On a more general note, anthropologist Anna Tsing draws on the analytical notion of a "commodity chain" when outlining how commodities transform as they move through different spheres and come to mean different things to different actors. Yet, Tsing points out, "the commodity must emerge as if untouched" (Tsing 2011:51).

As evident throughout the above empirical examples, the "life cycle" or "chain" through which pharmaceutical drugs had traveled before reaching the consumer in Egypt was not a theoretical argument or analytical tool, but an empirical reality. People in Cairo were thus very aware of the "chain" or different environments and contexts through which a pharmaceutical drug had traveled before it reached their hands (and bodies). The actual content of each link of the "chain" was left blurred, but the awareness of such links carrying the potential to affect and transform any given drug from its original form and intention was a very present experience: Where is this drug produced and by whom? How did it travel to Egypt? How did it travel within Egypt? Why this sudden shortage? Is this drug safe to take? Will it help or worsen my overall condition?

The above ethnographic encounter from Taher's workplace demonstrates these unresolved questions and uncertainties, and how they manifested in patients, for example, disrupting the intake of certain medicine based on their own immediate experiences or based on the advice of others besides their doctors. In addition, I might also mention here the uncertainty of the ways in which Taher was handing out medicine from his drawer – drugs that were no longer in a package and that could only be identified by size and color. According to Taher, the medicine had been donated by "some Swiss guy," but no one in the clinic really seemed to know for sure. I might also mention the uncertainty as to the women in front of the mosque who were vaccinating passer-byers, but according to Taher they were not affiliated with the clinic: he did not know who the women were, or where the vaccinations came from. Additionally, on our way to the clinic, Taher and I had passed a blood drive at one of the major metro stations in downtown Cairo. The blood drive was situated in the underground of the station, just off one of the platforms. Sunbeds were set up, and men were donating blood going in and out of the station. I poked Taher and asked him if maybe he should donate some blood – to which he simply responded (in a great summary of the above), "I don't know where these people are coming from, and I don't know where the blood is going." Taher noted that he did in fact donate blood regularly at the university hospital where he used to work – in what he considered to be a "much safer environment" for such an undertaking than the underground.

"Matter is always in movement, being molded and transformed by human and nonhuman processes and practices," I cited Hardon and Sanabria in the introduction to this chapter (Hardon and Sanabria 2017:118–19). As evident throughout this book thus far, this was not a theoretical argument, but an empirical realization among people in Cairo, both in relation to the consumption of food and beverages as outlined in the previous chapter, but also in relation to the consumption of pharmaceutical drugs. Politics, economies, corruption, environmental contaminations, and other global and local motions visibly affected the drug market in Egypt and the consumption of pharmaceutical drugs more specifically among the people that I was working with in Cairo during my fieldwork throughout the years of 2015–2017.

These motions were not invisible, or left as if "untouched," in the words of Tsing. Instead, people were acutely aware of the fact that pharmaceutical drugs were not drugs with objective intentions and forms. Rather, they could be molded and affected by a chain of people, places, environments, and politics, before finally reaching the hands and bodies of the consumer. This was a known fact, but one that generated a host of unknowns – unresolved questions regarding, for example, the agendas of people, companies, and governments, bribery and corruption, wrongful storage, expired expiration dates, counterfeit products, and so on. These fundamental uncertainties in turn left people generating uncertainties themselves, evident in the persistent reluctance and skepticism related to the intake of pharmaceutical drugs as prescribed by doctors, international guidelines, and pharmaceutical companies, all in an attempt to protect their bodies from potential harm.

Ahmed's Aunt Sums It Up (October 2015)

Ahmed's aunt greets us in the street. She kisses me on both cheeks and gives me her blessings. She is short, just like Ahmed's mother;

her dress drags along the ground, dirty and torn at the hem. We enter her small apartment, and sit beneath the harsh lights of two neon tubes. Ahmed's aunt looks sunburned and wrinkled from old age and life. She and Ahmed talk a lot and laugh a lot. I try my best to keep up with their conversation, but it's difficult. I look around and see wallpaper peeling off the walls, revealing quite a bit of mold underneath. Ahmed's aunt gets my attention and asks me if I want tea. Ahmed replies that we rather need something cold; we just had tea. He turns to me and asks if I would like some "*seven.*" 7-Up. I nod and tell him that "*seven*" would be nice. Ahmed and his aunt immediately jump from their chairs. They both want to go to the kiosk to buy "*seven.*" They literally argue for two minutes, both trying to slip their feet into the same flip-flops, pulling each other away from the door, back and forth, laughing at each other. Ahmed finally wins the battle, and leaves the apartment in a rush.

"He is a good boy," Ahmed's aunt concludes, satisfied.

Ahmed's aunt gets comfortable on the couch opposite me. She looks at me intensely for a couple of seconds, her eyes focused on mine. As I am getting ready to ask about her diabetes, she starts firing questions my way, almost shouting, presumably due to a hearing-impairment.

"ARE YOU MARRIED?" "DO YOU HAVE CHILDREN?" "WHY DO YOU NOT HAVE CHILDREN? IS SOMETHING WRONG WITH YOU? IS SOMETHING WRONG WITH YOUR HUSBAND?" "WHY DO YOU NOT VEIL? ARE YOU NOT A MUSLIM? WHAT ARE YOU?" I try to keep up with her questions. I finally reply that I am Christian, attempting a simple answer to a difficult question.

"*Rabina nafs, rabina nafs*, Our God is the same, our God is the same," Ahmed's aunt mumbles.

Ahmed returns from the kiosk and I feel relieved that he is back already. Ahmed's aunt immediately pours some *seven* for all of us. She starts talking about her children. She has four boys, and all of them are married.

"THEY LIVE IN HELIOPOLIS," she shouts, "far from here," she comments. "I like that they are far away, so I am far away from all of their problems," she says and laughs. She and Ahmed talk intensely about her children, Ahmed's cousins. I understand from the conversation that one of her sons is having problems with his wife. Or rather, perhaps, Ahmed's aunt is having a problem with the wife.

"I think he should take a new wife, but he says no," Ahmed's aunt explains. "She is always angry, she sits like this!" Ahmed's aunt starts shaking her whole body, making an angry face. "She needs to calm down," she adds.

"I told her that she should listen to her husband. I tried telling her this already," Ahmed says. Clearly, Ahmed and his aunt have discussed this issue before.

Ahmed's aunt suddenly looks at me.

"I have diabetes, that's why I have no teeth!" she says. She smiles, revealing a mouth of barely any teeth. I ask her if she sees a doctor regularly. She starts complaining about Egyptian doctors and hospitals.

"It's so much work, so much work," she says, explaining how visiting the doctor's office makes her "*taʿbāna gidan*, very tired." In fact, the trip to the doctor's office makes her feel worse than her diabetes in the first place. She starts explaining in detail the process of going to the doctor. First, she has to go to the lab to get her blood work done.

"And I am not allowed to eat anything before I go," she says. "At the lab, I have to pay someone to do their work properly," she further explains. She keeps elaborating how she then has to return to the lab on the following day to pick up her lab results, and then wait another day, before she can finally go to the diabetes clinic.

"At the clinic, I always have to wait the whole day, and also pay someone to do their work properly. Finally, I get to see the doctor, and he tells me I look tired, and that I am not taking good care of myself!" Ahmed and his aunt both laugh hysterically. "I am tired from running around and waiting in his office all day – not from my diabetes," she laughs. After a while, she finally adds, "So I stopped going, and I don't take my medicine either, and now I have no teeth." She cracks a big smile once again.

Treating the Present or the Future?

Dumit outlines how the past decades have marked a shift from a world in which pharmaceutical drugs were previously consumed primarily to treat current symptoms to a world today in which drugs are consumed primarily to prevent future symptoms (Dumit 2012:24). He outlines specifically how the introduction of clinical trials and mass statistics in the 1950s paved the way for newfound health notions such as "risk factors" and "chronic" conditions, notions pointing toward potential futures of late complications, as opposed to symptoms and ailments of the present (Dumit 2012:5–7). This is the case also of much diabetes medicine, which aims at controlling a present blood sugar in order to prevent future complications.

When Ahmed's aunt was initially diagnosed with type-2 diabetes she had primarily felt tired from the untreated high blood sugars. The metformin she was advised to take, however, had caused her to suffer from prolonged nausea and diarrhea. Thus, she stopped taking the pill, prioritizing her immediate experience of wellbeing, over medicating a potential future of late complications. One doctor coined this tendency among his patients to prioritize in such ways as Ahmed's aunt, "If they [the patients] wake up, and don't experience any symptoms of diabetes on that particular morning, they will simply skip an insulin treatment or change the dosage." He added, "They listen very little to what they should do."

I argue here that uncertainties related to the pharmaceutical industry as outlined throughout this chapter caused people in Cairo such as Ahmed's aunt and others to emphasize and trust primarily in their own present experiences of health and wellbeing over the advice and reassurances of doctors and pharmaceutical companies to attempt to maintain a certain future by the use of pharmaceutical drugs. Anthropologists Richard Jenkins, Hanne Jessen, and Vibeke Steffen have outlined how people "seek a sense of control when faced with crisis," including through seeking medical treatment and taking medicine when falling ill (Jenkins, Jessen, and Steffen 2005:9). However, based on the empirical examples presented throughout this chapter, I argue that to people in Cairo, taking pharmaceutical drugs, for example, to treat their type-2 diabetes, rather seemed to cause experiences of uncertainty and loss of control more than experiences of actually taking control. In many cases this caused people to make their own decisions and adjustments to the dosage of their medicine rather than taking the dosage advised by their doctors. In other cases, it meant a complete disruption of their treatment, such as in the above case of Ahmed's aunt, who decided that the symptoms and complications of her type-2 diabetes were less of a problem than the strain of enduring medical side effects and visiting the doctor's office ("I am tired from running around and waiting in his office all day – not from my diabetes," she insisted).

I want to stress here that uncertainties related to the consumption of pharmaceutical drugs did not prevent people in Cairo from treating ailments medically; however, most of the people that I came across maintained, disrupted, or adjusted their medicine intake first and foremost based on their own immediate experiences and the experiences of, for example, relatives as opposed to the advice given by doctors. This is evident in the previous empirical encounters in this chapter as well as in the cases of Taher's mother and aunt and in the cases of the two female patients consulting with Taher while he was working as a general practitioner. Here one young woman specifically expressed how a set of drugs given to her by the clinic – in her experience – did not work well on her body; rather, the drugs were making her feel worse ("My whole body is aching"). Taher firmly advised her against disrupting the treatment ("You should really keep taking these once you have started"), arguing that the woman's illness was making her feel ill, not the treatment itself ("You feel sick from your diarrhea, not from the medicine").

I do not know if that particular young woman stopped or continued her treatment, but I do know from many other medical consultations that I observed across various medical clinics in Cairo, as well as within all of the families that I was working with, that the possibility that she would defy Taher's advice was at least as likely as the possibility that she would follow his advice. Three of the people I knew really well within the families that I worked with in Cairo had, for example, chosen to completely end their treatment with metformin due to their own immediate negative experiences with the drug – despite the firm advice from their doctors to take the drug on a regular basis. This was the case of Ahmed's aunt as recounted above, as well as in the cases of one of Mohamed's aunts and of Mai's father (introduced in the following chapter). All three argued in similar ways as Ahmed's aunt that taking metformin had made them feel worse than their diabetes did in the first place.

Cast Your Vote Here (August 2015)

I enter the pharmacy to buy a few things; soap, chocolate, and chips. A girl in a school uniform enters. She is about 10 years old, and her hair is tied loosely on her head, strays of hair falling down along her face. A light blue bow hangs from her ponytail, untied; it appears to be part of the school uniform. She is wearing oversized jeans and a big school backpack. She tugs at her jeans while strolling around the pharmacy, with a stick in her right hand, picking out a bag of chips. She is quietly whistling a song. Suddenly the pharmacist, an elderly man, yells: "*ISTAGHFAR ALLĀH!* I seek forgiveness from Allah. GIRLS DON'T WHISTLE!" he shouts. The girl grabs a bag of chips and looks at the man. She angrily whistles back at him, "FWEEEET!" The man raises his hands as if he is about to slap the girl. "I WILL TELL YOUR FATHER!" he shouts. The girl throws a pound on the counter and runs out of the pharmacy. I am looking around, a bit puzzled as to what just happened. I quickly pay for my soaps and chocolates, and as I leave the pharmacy, I see the girl quietly walking down the street, hitting her stick on the ground as she goes. A younger boy suddenly jumps out from a doorway and screams, "YOUR FATHER IS A GARBAGE MAN!" The girl turns around and chases after the boy, stick in the air.

I get in a taxi. We cross Tahrir Square. I roll down the window; it's hot and dusty. The square is decorated with lights, flags, and big inflatable bears. A giant Egyptian flag is hanging from the top of the Mugamma, a major administrative building. It's covering most of the building, reaching almost all the way to the ground. The city is getting ready for the festivities of the grand opening of the new Suez Canal. There is a big banner in the middle of the square. It reads in English, "EGYPT'S GIFT TO THE WORLD." I consider whether or not I should participate in the festivities. The taxi driver is quiet as we go. I observe the city as we leave downtown on one of the expressways above the smaller streets. Egyptian flags and balloons are everywhere, not only in Tahrir Square.

There is a lot of traffic on the way, and for a while we come to a standstill. I study some graffiti on a wall – a stick figure is putting a piece of paper in a trash bin. "Cast your vote here," it says above the figure.

The taxi driver turns on the radio. The hosts are debating the canal. Whether it can be considered "new" at all. The debate is interrupted by commercials, and a particular radio spot, advertising the expansion of the canal. A deep, soft, female voice speaks, "*Min ʾumm il-dunyā li kul il-dunyā*, From the mother of the world to the whole world." We stop at a red light. Suddenly a mob of men, fists held tight, pass in between the cars. The taxi sways from side to side as the men push their way through. They are all marching in the same direction, shouting something in unison. They look angry. The taxi driver looks at them in the rear-view mirror as our stop-light turns green and we speed away.

Summary

In this chapter, I have extended the arguments of the previous chapters by depicting the ways in which a reluctance to take metformin among some of the people I met in Cairo stemmed in part from an overall resistance to accept the etiology of "diabesity." The potential effect of metformin to induce a weight loss was, in other words, considered an illegitimate target of type-2 diabetes treatment; metformin thus was not a desirable drug. Additionally, uncertainties related to the general intake of pharmaceutical drugs caused concerns over the actual workings of metformin and what was perceived as its potential to damage the kidneys. Overall, I have shown how uncertainties related to the pharmaceutical industry and to the "life cycle" (Geest, Hardon, and Whyte 1996:171) of pharmaceutical drugs caused the people that I worked with in Cairo to emphasize personal medical experiences and the medical experiences of, for example, relatives above the advice and reassurances of doctors and medical companies as to the workings of specific drugs. This additionally added to the potential disruption of taking, for example, metformin, as the side effects of this particular drug to some were experienced as worse than the symptoms of type-2 diabetes in the first place.

Overall, this chapter has discussed the ways in which the pharmaceutical industry enhances a neoliberal understanding of type-2 diabetes in its attempts to medicate individual bodies and their supposed obesity. As depicted throughout the above, people in Cairo were reluctant to merely accept the idea of "diabesity"; first, aware of the ways in which type-2 diabetes in their perspective was rather related to experiences of *ḍaghṭ* caused by a great many uncertainties in many spheres of everyday life, and, second, as the supply and use of pharmaceutical drugs were so evidently linked to such uncertainties in the first place – adding to experiences of *ḍaghṭ* and thus to the potential onset and worsening of type-2 diabetes. This chapter serves as a critical reminder that to people in Cairo type-2 diabetes treatment was not simply a matter of losing weight and taking metformin, but a matter of a great many other structural conditions; conditions best, perhaps, treated elsewhere than within individual bodies.

Note

1 15 EGP was equivalent to approximately 0.8 USD as of October 2018.

References

Dumit, Joseph. 2012. *Drugs for Life: How Pharmaceutical Companies Define Our Health*. Duke University Press.

El-Fekki, Amira. 2015. Dehydrated Infants Die in Hospital of Faulty Drugs: Health Ministry. July 27, 2015. Daily News Egypt. https://dailynewsegypt.com/2015/07/27/dehydrated-infants-die-in-hospital-of-faulty-drugs-health-ministry/.

Geest, Sjaak van der, Anita Hardon, and Susan R. Whyte. 1996. The Anthropology of Pharmaceuticals: A Biographical Approach. *Annual Review of Anthropology* 25(1): 153–178.

Glasgow, Sara, and Ted Schrecker. 2016. The Double Burden of Neoliberalism? Noncommunicable Disease Policies and the Global Political Economy of Risk. *Health & Place* 39: 204–211.

Hardon, Anita, and Emilia Sanabria. 2017. Fluid Drugs: Revisiting the Anthropology of Pharmaceuticals. *Annual Review of Anthropology* 46: 117–132.

Heine, R. J., M. Diamant, J. C. Mbanya, and D. M. Nathan. 2006. Management of Hyperglycaemia in Type 2 Diabetes: The End of Recurrent Failure? *British Medical Journal* 333(7580): 1200–1204.

Hunt, Linda. 2017. How Big Business Is Re-Defining Illness and Health: Fabrication of a Block Buster Drug Market. *In* Conference of the Australian Anthropological Society and the Association of Social Anthropologists. Adelaide Australia.

Inzucchi, S. E., K. J. Lipska, H. Mayo, C. J. Bailey, and D. K. McGuire. 2014. Metformin in Patients with Type 2 Diabetes and Kidney Disease: A Systematic Review. *JAMA* 312(24): 2668–2675.

Jenkins, Richard, Hanne Jessen, and Vibeke Steffen. 2005. Matters of Life and Death: The Control of Uncertainty and the Uncertainty of Control. *In Managing Uncertainty: Ethnographic Studies of Illness, Risk and the Struggle for Control.* Richard Jenkins, Hanne Jessen, and Vibeke Steffen, eds. Pp. 9–29. Museum Tusculanum.

Jöhncke, Steffen, Mette Nordahl Svendsen, and Susan Reynolds Whyte. 2004. Løsningsmodeller: Sociale Teknologier Som Antropologisk Arbejdsfelt. *In Viden Om Verden.* Kirsten Hastrup, ed. Pp. 385–407. Hans Reitzel.

Landecker, Hannah. 2016. Antibiotic Resistance and the Biology of History. *Body & Society* 22(4): 19–52.

Lupton, Deborah. 2013. *Fat.* Routledge.

Nading, Alex M. 2017. Local Biologies, Leaky Things, and the Chemical Infrastructure of Global Health. *Medical Anthropology* 36(2): 141–156.

Nye, Helen J., and William G. Herrington. 2011. Metformin: The Safest Hypoglycaemic Agent in Chronic Kidney Disease? *Nephron Clinical Practice* 118(4): 380–383.

Petryna, Adriana, and Arthur Kleinman. 2006. The Pharmaceutical Nexus. *In Global Pharmaceuticals: Ethics, Markets, Practices.* Adriana Petryna, Andrew Lakoff, and Arthur Kleinman, eds. Pp. 1–32. Duke University Press.

Phillips, Tarryn, Celia McMichael, and Michael O'Keefe. 2018. "We Invited the Disease to Come to Us": Neoliberal Public Health Discourse and Local Understanding of Non-Communicable Disease Causation in Fiji. *Critical Public Health* 28(5): 560–572.

Rajan, Kaushik Sunder. 2017. *Pharmocracy: Value, Politics, and Knowledge in Global Biomedicine.* Duke University Press.

Reubi, David, Clare Herrick, and Tim Brown. 2016. The Politics of Non-Communicable Diseases in the Global South. *Health & Place* 39: 179–187.

Sismondo, Sergio. 2015. Pushing Knowledge in the Drug Industry: Ghost-Managed Science. *In The Pharmaceutical Studies Reader*. S. Sismondo, and J. Greene, eds. Pp. 150–164. Wiley Blackwell.

Spector, Malcolm, and John I. Kitsuse. 2001. *Constructing Social Problems*. Transaction Publishers.

Tawfeek, Farah. 2017. Ex-President of State-Owned Drug Company Faces Imprisonment for Causing Penicillin Shortage Crisis. December 20 2017. Egypt Independent. www.egyptindependent.com/ex-president-of-state-owned-drug-company-faces-imprisonment-for-causing-penicillin-shortage-crisis/.

Trnka, Susanna, and Catherine Trundle. 2017. *Competing Responsibilities: The Politics and Ethics of Contemporary Life*. Susanna Trnka, and Catherine Trundle, eds. Duke University Press.

Tsing, Anna L. 2011. *Friction: An Ethnography of Global Connection*. Princeton University Press.

Wanis, Heba. 2015. Pharmaceutical Pricing in Egypt. *In Pharmaceutical Prices in the 21st Century*. Zaheer-Ud-Din Babar, ed. Pp. 59–78. Springer.

Wilson, Elizabeth A. 2015. *Gut Feminism*. Duke University Press.

5 Care

Literature within the field of medical anthropology has addressed the role of nonprofessional caregivers in the task of caring for the ill. The literature particularly stresses the "work" that is required to manage chronic illnesses at home (see, for example, Mattingly, Grøn, and Meinert 2011; Mol 2008), as well as the "moral task" of caring for ill family members (Kleinman 2009). Anthropologist Hayder al-Mohammad has argued that it takes the "struggle" of many to sustain the life of one. From his work in Iraq he argues, "It is because life can be something in jeopardy, pain, threatened, or taken away that the wounding and suffering of others [...] can be felt so directly by those whose lives are enmeshed and intertwined with theirs" (Al-Mohammad 2012:608). For these reasons, he argues, loved ones may undertake great personal struggles to maintain the lives of others (Al-Mohammad 2012:600).

I now turn to address the ways in which type-2 diabetes treatment within the families that I was working with in Cairo aimed at relieving the diabetic body of experiences of *ḍaghṭ* as opposed to adding additional *ḍaghṭ*, for example, by implementing a strict diet and physical exercise or by measuring blood sugars meticulously. Caring for family members with type-2 diabetes, instead, revolved around relieving the ill of pressures of everyday life, for example, by relieving them of going to the market, bargaining their way from vendor to vendor, but also by keeping them away from stressful news or conditions within the family. However, relieving family members of such pressures did not simply make these pressures go away; rather, I argue, they shifted from the person diagnosed with type-2 diabetes to the relatives involved in their care, essentially placing those relatives at risk of developing type-2 diabetes themselves.

In this chapter, I recount one such struggle of a young woman, Mai, in her late 20s, who had lost her mother due to complications

DOI: 10.4324/9781003327684-5

of type-2 diabetes prior to my fieldwork in Cairo, and whose father was very ill from type-2 diabetes when I arrived in the city in 2015. Both the death of Mai's mother and the current condition of her father affected Mai's life and wellbeing greatly. This became evident in the ways that she and her older sister, Reem, handled another vulnerable situation within the family: their older brother falling ill with schizophrenia. In the first part of the chapter, I explain how Mai struggled to endure her role as a loved one caring for the health of both her father and brother. Drawing on Al-Mohammed, I argue that the lives of the individuals I came across in Cairo were greatly intertwined with the lives of their family members as the choices and behaviors of one greatly affected those of others.

In the second part of the chapter, I show how Mai's attempts to relieve her father and brother of the pressures of everyday life did not make these pressures go away; rather, they shifted to Mai and her sister. Thus, I argue, type-2 diabetes came to affect not only the bodies of those diagnosed with the condition, but also the bodies of those who were involved in their care. Overall, I draw on the arguments of anthropologist Amy Moran-Thomas and others to dissolve the dualism of communicable/non-communicable conditions and the popular framing of, for example, type-2 diabetes as a non-communicable disease. Moran-Thomas instead proposes the notion of "para-communicable" conditions to capture the ways in which conditions such as type-2 diabetes arguably "spread" and one may "catch" the condition (Moran-Thomas 2019a). Similarly, I wish to finally point to the ways in which type-2 diabetes spread through the city of Cairo, including within intimate relations in family households.

Ḥāsbī! Careful! (August 2015)

The tips of Mai's scarf blow in the wind. The scarf is tied neatly around her hair; her hair fixed in a bun at the back of her head. Her neck is bare. A few black hairs are visible from underneath her scarf. Mai is looking up and down the street with a careless gaze. She looks exhausted, moving her body slowly. She moves her head left, then right, before moving her feet forward, then backwards again. Her arm slowly touches my chest and stops me from crossing the street as a car passes by at high speed.

Mai's older sister, Reem, is full of energy, laughing and chattering away. It's nighttime in Heliopolis, and we are trying to cross a busy street. Reem is throwing popcorn at me while lightheartedly telling me about a man who wants to marry her.

"Careful, Reem … *Ḥāsbī*," Mai says, trying to get us safely across the street.

"He is a dentist," Reem says. "Or we call him *the butcher*," she laughs. We quickly cross the street, dodging traffic and crossing old tram tracks.

"We met him at his office," Reem explains energetically. "Mai had a tooth-problem." Mai is ignoring Reem, scouting the street for cafes. Reem continues, "He took a very long time extracting the tooth … asking me to assist during the surgery … as if I was his nurse!" Reem laughs at the story. "That's why we call him *the butcher*."

We walk down one of the big boulevards. It's dark, yet the streets are flooded with lights from the colorful shop windows; clothes, chocolates, balloons, teddy bears, handbags, coffee, honey, shoes, laughter. Big smiles. Reem continues the story, "Later, he came to our house to propose to me. *Baba* didn't like him, but that's okay, we didn't really like him either." Mai stops in the middle of the sidewalk, Reem and I follow suit. Reem makes a face, as she mocks the dentist's name, "Faauwzziiii …" Reem and I both laugh. "It's a very old name," she says, adding, "I want someone named Mohamed or Ahmed. Those are good and strong names."

Mai points to a sidewalk café in an alley behind us. "Maybe here is good?" she asks. We nod, and grab a couple of plastic chairs, arranging them and ourselves around one of the available coffee tables. Reem has a playful smile, as if she is about to tell us something funny. Mai is studying the menu.

"I want to marry myself," Reem then suddenly declares. Mai looks up from the menu. I turn my head and look at Reem. "Yes, I want to marry myself!" she says again. I laugh, Mai rolls her eyes. "They do it in Hollywood," Reem says, shrugging her shoulders. After a while she says, "I pray to Allah to make me free and let me leave the house."

"*ʾIn shāʾ allāh*, God willing," Mai mumbles.

I quickly mumble an "*ʾin shāʾ allāh*" as well.

I ask Reem what happened to her fiancé, the one she was engaged to a while back. The doctor.

"I broke it off, he was very materialistic. He wanted me to work and give him all of my money. If I married him, I would be like any Egyptian woman. Not happy," Reem says.

"Really *Mila*, there was a lot of pressure for Reem to marry this man. *Ḍaghṭ kathīr*. A lot of pressure. From our father, from our brother, and from the sheikh," Mai jumps in. Mai abruptly changes the topic, and asks if we want pasta and Pepsi. We both nod. She gets up to order. Reem immediately turns to me, and speaks in a low voice.

"I do not want to talk about anything bad when Mai returns. She has been very depressed now for almost two years. Sometimes she doesn't eat or sleep or speak to anyone for weeks." Reem is speaking rapidly. Mai quickly returns to the table.

"Are you talking about me behind my back?" she asks.

"Yes," we answer in unison.

We try to keep the conversation light while eating our pasta. I ask Mai about her upcoming exams and her work as a tour guide.

"My first tour was during the revolution. I was so scared. You know, everything closed down because of the demonstrations. My first tour and I get stuck in a hotel with five strange men for three days!" We all laugh.

"After that experience everything else must have seemed easy," I tell Mai.

"No, I wish," Mai responds.

We sit quietly for a while. Mai then asks the waiter if they have ice cream.

"We have very good pasta," he responds. We laugh.

"We just had pasta," Mai says. We pay for our food and move toward McDonald's across the street.

"They have ice cream," Mai says.

We enter the fast-food restaurant. It looks the same as in any other city around the world. Only a few posters of the Pyramids and the Karnak Temple indicate that we are in Egypt. The Ronald McDonald clown has been photoshopped into the pictures. The restaurant is full of families and the acoustics are really bad. We quickly pick up some ice cream at the counter and sit at one of the few available tables. Mai eats a spoonful of ice cream.

"Reem and I are seeing a psychologist," Mai says. Reem shushes Mai. Reem lowers her voice while looking around at people in our close vicinity.

"It's *our* secret that we are seeing a psychologist," she says.

"There is nothing wrong with seeing a psychologist," Mai responds at a normal volume. I ask the two why they are seeing a psychologist.

"Because of my depression," Mai says.

"Because we both have a complex with men," Reem says. She explains that they are seeing a male psychologist. "It's the first time I have ever cried in front of a man," she whispers. "He is like a mother to me."

Mai interrupts, "I call him *Baba*, Reem calls him *Mama*." We all laugh.

Family Ties (Introducing Mai)

I first met Mai and her sister Reem in 2010 when I was studying Arabic in Cairo. On returning to Cairo in 2015 to conduct the first phase of fieldwork for this book, I reached out to the girls, remembering that their father had type-2 diabetes. The girls quickly agreed to help me with my research, including sharing their own story. As it turned out, the girls had lost their mother to a type-2 diabetes-related stroke in 2008, more specifically due to many years of living with a poorly regulated blood sugar. At the time of my fieldwork in Cairo in 2015, the father of Mai and Reem was also very ill from type-2 diabetes. Due to late complications of his condition, he had gone almost completely blind in both eyes, and was struggling with foot ulcers, leaving him at great risk of infections and potential amputations. The girls lived with their father on the outskirts of Heliopolis in the northeastern part of Cairo in a two-bedroom apartment along the metro tracks.

The family had moved to Cairo from a village in the northern part of Egypt after the passing of their mother, allowing the girls to attend university in the city. Mai, Reem, and their father did not live near their extended family, unlike most of the other families that I knew in Cairo. The girls also had an older brother, Sherif, who was working in Sinai, about a day's travel from Cairo. He rarely came to visit his father and sisters, but when he did come for a visit, the girls did not speak of him fondly. "He is such a monster," Reem said. "He is like a dictator," Mai would chime in, complaining that he would interfere with the way they dressed and the hours they spent outside of their home.

At the time of my fieldwork in 2015, both girls had graduated from college, and were well on their way to establishing their careers, Mai within tourism and Reem within therapy and private coaching. "We attract work and money easily, but not men," Mai summed up their lives. Naturally, the passing of their mother had left the girls in much grief, but also in a social limbo of a sort. In Egypt, it is often the role of the mother (and of other female kin) to assist their daughters and sons in finding a suitable spouse (see also Ghannam 2013). Since the girls had neither their mother, nor any other female kin close by, their father, brother, and local sheikh had taken on the social responsibility of getting the girls married. So far, in vain.

At the time of my fieldwork in 2015, the girls were in their late 20s and early 30s, already considered old for marriage by some. Sherif, their older brother, had declared that he would not marry himself until both of the girls had married; being the only son, he was financially responsible for the family, and if his father were to pass away, he would be legally responsible for his sisters as well (until they were married). He explained that he did not want to take on the responsibility of a family of his own, as long as he was still responsible for his father and his two sisters.

The girls were very vocal about their desires to find a suitable husband. Both yearned for "*ḥubb*, love," and to be able to leave their father's house and establish a family of their own. Yet, at the time of the above empirical encounter, both girls were fed up with what was in their perspectives bad proposals (from men similar to "the butcher"), and with the *ḍaghṭ* inflicted on them by both their brother and father and local sheikh to marry men of their choosing (such as "the doctor"). Reem thus declared partly joking, partly serious, "I want to marry myself," while Mai was showing increasingly worrisome signs of depression. "We both have a complex with men," Reem announced, summing up the consequences of past encounters with prospective husbands, as well as the involvement of their father and brother in these encounters.

Due to these past experiences, both girls had come to insist that they would marry out of love, not out of practicalities or due to pressures put on them by their father, brother, or by others. "First love, then marriage," Mai often stated, contrary to the usual process among many of the people that I knew in Cairo of "first marriage, then love." Maha, for example, often explained that assessing a man for marriage was primarily a matter of assessing if one could *potentially* love the man. In other words, Maha and others expected love to flourish in a marriage, but most (particularly those who were already married) acknowledged that initial feelings of love were not necessary before an engagement, as long as there was a potential for love to grow in the course of the marriage. Reem and Mai did not feel this way at all. They firmly expressed that they expected love to grow before they would ever agree to an engagement.

In fact, Maha had voiced somewhat the same opinion before finally agreeing to marry her cousin, Mustafa. As described in Chapter 3, Maha actually met with 11 suitors before finally settling for Mustafa. Throughout this process, her mother, aunts, sister, and female cousins had put a lot of effort into pushing Maha toward her cousin, raising the exact question posed by Maha in the above – whether she could *potentially* love him. In the first months of their engagement, Maha often confided in me that she "still" did not love Mustafa, but this had all finally changed by the time that I stayed with them at the beginning of my fieldwork in 2015. By then their story had turned into a love story of sorts, and love and marriage had merged in the mind of Maha. Maha happily emphasized how Mustafa had not inquired about other girls in the process prior to their engagement. Only she had felt uncertain, while he had patiently waited for her to decide. To Maha, this was true love.

Maha, Mai, and Reem were not alone in their approaches to love, as most of the men and women that I spoke to on this particular topic mentioned similar dilemmas or reflections. From his work in Egypt, anthropologist Samuli Schielke has also outlined how most young Egyptians (men and women) have ideas of love that relate to notions of both romance and desire, as well as to chastity and parental control over marriage (Schielke 2009:31). He writes, "The attempt to combine love and marriage [...] is an attempt to combine two languages that not only follow different grammars but also communicate different things" (Schielke 2015:95). In the case of Mai and Reem, this was very clear; the two ways of approaching love and marriage expressed by their father and brother and by themselves, respectively, did not apply the same "grammar." Rather, the girls argued, the two approaches to love and marriage were incompatible. Similar to Mai and Reem, their brother expressed how the girls were putting a lot of *ḍaghṭ* on him by their resistance to marry, even men of financially stable backgrounds (Reem proclaiming in the above that such "materialistic" men would merely make her feel like "any other Egyptian woman ... not happy"). In other words, the girls and their brother were tied together in a kind of deadlock, affecting the wellbeing and life paths of each other greatly.

I emphasize this story of love here to illustrate the ways in which individual lives interconnect greatly in families in Egypt. Drawing on Al-Mohammad's arguments presented in the introduction to this chapter (Al-Mohammad 2012), I argue along the same lines here that individual lives among the families that I was working with in Cairo were tied to or intertwined with the common life project of the family as a whole (for similar arguments from within an Egyptian context see, for example, Ghannam 2013; Hamdy 2012). Al-Mohammad argues, "We are not dealing with two lives but two different movements directed towards the one life project" (Al-Mohammad 2010:438). For these reasons, in Cairo as well, the choices and behaviors of one family member would greatly affect the choices and opportunities of the others. This was particularly evident in the case of love and marriage within Mai's family, as the fact that the girls were holding off on marrying affected their brother's ability to establish a family of his own. It was also evident in the circumstance that the death of their mother had left their father and brother with the unfamiliar task of preparing the girls for marriage.

I do not know if Mai and Reem's perspective on love and marriage would have been different had their mother been alive, but I do know from other cases of young women from similar backgrounds as the girls (such as Maha) that mothers and other female kin play an important role in preparing (or grooming) women for marriage. This often includes reversing notions of "first love, then marriage," and doing so patiently (for example, by going through 11 suitors as in Maha's case). In the case of Mai and Reem, their father, brother, and local sheikh appeared not to understand the importance of this time-consuming process of preparation and guidance – or maybe they did, but they did not know how to approach it. As a result, the girls felt rushed and pushed into meeting with potential suitors, as well as misunderstood when declining marriage.

A couple of weeks following the aforementioned night out with Mai and Reem, I received a text message from the girls stating that their brother, Sherif, had been admitted to the hospital. According to the text message, Sherif had suffered "a psychological shock." Upon seeing the girls, I learned that Reem had received a phone call from one of Sherif's colleagues, explaining that Sherif had shown up for work, but with a sudden change in behavior and personality. He had first insisted that his name was Sammy, not Sherif, and that he was an officer working for the Egyptian secret police. He had then punched a colleague, and turned to punch himself, upon which he had run out of the office and attempted suicide by drowning in the sea. Colleagues had pulled him out of the water, and taken him to a nearby hospital.

At first, the doctors had suspected a neurological disorder; however, all of the tests came back negative. Instead, Sherif was moved to a psychiatric hospital in Cairo where he was later diagnosed with schizophrenia. The girls explained that Sherif had not recognized either of them when they came to visit him in the hospital. Rather, he had claimed that he had no sisters. Sherif had not been able to leave his bed for weeks without assistance from the nurses, weak from his condition and from being heavily medicated. When I asked the girls about their father, they told me that they were keeping the hospitalization, and their brother's diagnosis, a secret from him.

"He has diabetes and high blood pressure," Reem argued, "I am sure the *ḍagḥṭ*, pressure of everything that happened to Sherif will make him really sick. I am scared to tell him."

Why Should I Care? (September 2015)

Reem sings an old Arabic song, her voice soft and deep. "*ʾAnā mālī wa ʾanā mālī?* Why should I care? Why should I care?"[1] she sings. The sun is setting, and the bats are starting to come out. Reem, Mai, three of their girlfriends, and I are sitting in a park in the middle of Cairo, enjoying the early evening breeze. We are sitting in a closed circle, with tea, soda cans, and sweets spread out between us. Our shoes are in a pile behind me, with our bare feet touching the grass. Some of the girls have closed their eyes, listening intensely to Reem singing. It sounds beautiful. I close my eyes as well.

Suddenly the girls start clapping and singing along. "*Wa bʾaḥibbak ʿawī ya ʿayūnī*, I love you so much, through my whole being." We all laugh. After a while, Reem stops singing and starts handing out tea. We all sit quietly for a while, enjoying the silence and the cooling weather. Mai breaks the silence.

"Our doctor, the psychologist, loves Reem," she says. Reem laughs and hides her face behind her hands.

Mai continues, "He sent me a really formal text message and Reem a really sweet message. I told Reem, 'Don't you see how different these messages are?' Reem didn't think so. A week later, he asked Reem if she had not noticed that he has feelings for her. She said 'No, but Mai has!'" Everyone laughs. "We are not going back there!" Mai declares, sipping from her tea.

One of the girls asks about Sherif, how he is doing. Reem says, "He is really weak. The nurse had to hold his hand around the ward yesterday." Mai comments, "I had a *breakdown* at the hospital," using the English word "breakdown." Reem nods, and then explains how Sherif kept crying out in the hospital, "I want to get married. I want to get married." She looks into her cup of tea, and adds, "But he doesn't want to marry till after Mai and I marry." The other girls nod silently. Someone says something encouraging and pats Reem's knee. Mai says that she is afraid she and Reem made Sherif sick, "because Reem didn't want to marry that doctor, and I also did not like the one he presented to me." Mai adds, "I also asked him to call someone to help me with something work-related … I think it was too much to ask of him." Reem says, "I am going to work really hard so he doesn't have to worry about us." One of the girls says that she thinks Reem and Mai are really "brave."

Reem changes the topic. She instructs us all to lie on our backs and look up at the starlit sky. She tells us to bend our legs, so our feet are touching the ground. It's good for our "health" to stay "grounded" in nature, she says, using the English words "health" and "grounded." Bats are flying around above our heads. We all lie there quietly for a while. Reem breaks the silence, "Every day I sit on the balcony, and pray, and speak to Allah. Yesterday he spoke back to me. He told me, don't worry. Be safe. It will be okay."

After a while, we gather our things and walk toward the exit. Mai and I linger behind the other girls. Mai takes my arm and interlocks it with hers. I ask her how she is doing. "I am really sad," she says. I nod my head. The other girls pass a young boy on a bench in front of us. He is singing an Arabic pop-song, while his friend is filming him with a cell phone. Reem and one of the other girls crack up laughing. I can hear Reem say, "He has such a girly voice. I want a man with a real man voice."

Shifting Pressures

When falling ill, Sherif had gone from a "monster" and a "dictator," in the perspective of his sisters, to a "weak" young man in desperate need of love and care. Sherif's newfound condition illustrated that, of course, there was more to the relationship between him and his sisters than mutual pressure. "Why should I care?" Reem sings poetically in the above, perhaps providing the answer herself in the following as well – because "I love you through my whole being." In the weeks following Sherif's hospitalization, the girls visited their brother as often as the healthcare personnel would allow it. They would hold his hand, sing to him, sit quietly in the room, and wait for him to get better. Both girls were speculating a lot about the reasons for his condition, as well as possible treatments and the prospects of his wellbeing. They were very concerned about their roles in relation to the onset of his illness, particularly how their resistance to marrying had left him with a prolonged financial burden and the inability to start his own family.

Sherif's condition drove Reem to work even harder than she had done before his hospitalization. Prior to her brother falling ill, she had strived toward financial independence from her father and brother, primarily as a way to position herself better in case she needed to resist marrying someone she did not like. After Sherif's hospitalization, she rather strived toward financial independence as a way to relieve her brother of the financial pressure of taking care of her and Mai (and of their father as well). Reem was convinced that such financial relief would leave their brother in a better general state, as well as allow him to settle and initiate a family of his own, something he clearly desired ("I want to get married, I want to get married," Reem recounted his outbursts in the hospital). "Falling in love," Reem argued, would in fact be the best treatment of all. Working hard also allowed Reem to pay bills that were normally paid by her brother – and thus to keep Sherif's hospitalization hidden from their father. This was necessary, Reem argued, to protect their father's health by not adding additional "*ḍaghṭ*" to his already fragile body.

Mai reacted to Sherif's situation differently than Reem. At the time of our above visit to the park, Mai had gradually begun to question her own convictions of "first love, then marriage." Shortly after our night out at the park, she had reached out to a man previously presented to her by her brother. "Maybe I can learn to love him," she argued, though she quickly cut it off with the man, finally stating, "The idea of marrying him makes me feel miserable." At the time, Mai's depressed mental state was manifesting itself physically. Shortly after our night out at the park, she was, in fact, diagnosed with hypertension, high blood pressure. In addition, she was shredding chunks of hair, and her body was breaking out in a sudden rash. Her doctor was unable to explain the latter two conditions, but advised Mai to take antihypertensive medication and to rest. Mai herself was certain; she was suffering from "*il-ḍaghṭ*," both literally (hypertension), but also in more general terms (from pressures of everyday life).

I argue here that the intertwinements of individual lives into the one life project of the family caused a shifting of *ḍaghṭ* from family members to others and thus carried the risk of potentially transmitting the condition of type-2 diabetes within the families that I was working with in Cairo. This was evident, for example, in the ways Maha and others relieved their family members diagnosed with type-2 diabetes from going to the market and the like; or in the ways Mai and Reem took it upon themselves to keep the condition of their brother a secret from their father. Such attempts at relieving family members diagnosed with type-2 diabetes of various sorts of pressures were driven by a concern as to the ways in which experiences of *ḍaghṭ* might worsen the condition of type-2 diabetes.

However, such experiences of *ḍaghṭ* did not go away through these acts of care, but rather shifted to Maha, Mai, Reem, and others, as they themselves were left experiencing "*ḍaghṭ kathīr*, a lot of pressure" from the tasks undertaken in their endeavors to take proper care of their loved ones. This left them not only experiencing "*ḍaghṭ kathīr*," but also with physiological manifestations of such *ḍaghṭ*, evident, for example, in the swelling of Maha's pregnant body and in Mai's condition of hypertension. Reem worked incredibly hard to make ends meet financially upon her brother falling ill, and shortly after the above-outlined trip to the park she acknowledged the "*ḍaghṭ*" that her brother must have felt to sustain the family. Mai, on the other hand, strongly reconsidered marriage to a man she did not love in order to permanently relieve her brother (as well as her father and sister) of the "*ḍaghṭ*" of taking care of her financially. Mai, in other words, felt the pressure of finding a husband more than ever.

Recent work within medical anthropology has aimed to dissolve the biomedical distinction between "communicable" and "non-communicable" conditions, arguing that so-called "non-communicable diseases" (such as type-2 diabetes) may, in fact, be considered "communicable," even if they are not infectious in a biological sense (see, for example, Christensen and Seeberg 2017; Grøn 2017; Nielsen 2017; Seeberg and Meinert 2015). Anthropologists Lotte Meinert and Jens Seeberg, for example, have proposed to explore ways in which conditions such as type-2 diabetes are contagious locally through biosocial relations and networks. They encourage raising the question, "What is transmitted and how?" (Seeberg and Meinert 2015:62). Similarly, anthropologist Amy Moran-Thomas has proposed the use of the notion "para-communicable" in relation to conditions "materially transmitted as bodies and ecologies intimately shape each other over time, with unequal and compounding effects for historically situated groups of people" (Moran-Thomas 2019a:497).

Throughout the book thus far, I have aimed to outline how type-2 diabetes in the perspective of those diagnosed with the condition, as well as in the perspective of many of their relatives, was considered to transmit through the streets of Cairo. *Ḍaghṭ*, I have shown, was caused by a plethora of conditions related to structural factors of great uncertainties, manifested, for example, in sudden shifts in the economy, the possible consumption of poisonous foods and questionable medications, or the risk of exposing oneself to medical misconduct in general. In this chapter specifically, I have additionally outlined how *ḍaghṭ*, as a factor of transmission, may shift from the person who is diagnosed with type-2 diabetes to his or her family members through acts of care, potentially causing type-2 diabetes to transmit within families.

Moran-Thomas has argued from her work on diabetes in Belize, "Communicability is not just a matter of seeing and interpreting the causes of disease, but also a factor shaping the plausibility and workability of treatment" (Moran-Thomas 2019b:475). Extending the arguments from the previous chapters here, I once again wish to question the ways in which certain treatment and prevention strategies foregrounding an etiology of "diabesity" were promoted in relation to type-2 diabetes in Egypt in the years of 2015–2017, largely overlooking the ways in which structural conditions, as well as intimate relations and intertwinements within families, arguably carried the risk of transmitting type-2 diabetes.

Mohamed Is Really Osama (February 2017)

"Wait for me outside. I am coming!" Mohamed says on the phone. I hang up and look around the streets. I am in downtown Cairo in front of the office building of a public newspaper. Mohamed occasionally works here, and we are meeting up to go visit his mother. The office building is large. The other side of the street is full of small kiosks and coffee shops, catering to all the workers in the area.

"You are not allowed to stand here," a man suddenly says in Arabic. I turn around and face a security officer. He looks angry as he repeats, "You are not allowed to stand here. It's forbidden, *mamnūʿ*." He doesn't give me time to answer, but immediately follows up, "What are you doing here?" I try to find the right words in Arabic, but I suddenly feel caught off-guard. It makes me nervous. I try explaining that I am waiting for someone who works inside the building. Another security officer quickly joins us. "You are not allowed to stand here," he says in Arabic as well. "It's forbidden," he adds. I try explaining in Arabic that I am meeting someone who works at the newspaper. The first officer tells me that I have to wait inside the building. "You are not allowed to wait out here," he repeats, and points me toward the entrance.

I leave the officers behind and quickly walk toward the entrance of the building. I feel the officers staring me down. Another security officer stops me at the entrance. "What do you want? *ʿAyza ayh*?" he snaps at me. I tell him that I am waiting for a friend who works here. "You are not allowed to wait inside," the officer tells me and points me toward the exit. I explain that the officers outside just told me that I have to wait inside the building.

"Who are you waiting for?" he asks.

"Mohamed ..." I reply, trying to think of Mohamed's last name, but in vain.

"Everyone here is named Mohamed," the officer replies, irritated. "Mohamed who?" he asks. I tell him that I forgot Mohamed's last name. Perhaps I can try to call him on my phone. I try to call Mohamed, but he doesn't pick up and I start to feel a bit desperate. The officer shakes his head and points me toward the chairs in the middle of the hall. I sit down, nervously looking up the stairs and at the elevators, hoping for Mohamed to appear.

I occasionally glance over at the officer, who seems to be watching me in return. After a while, Mohamed finally appears from the elevators. I get up to greet him, with great relief. We quickly exit the building and pass the officers outside on our way. I try not to look at them, but Mohamed greets them. One of the officers quickly apologizes to Mohamed. "I didn't know you knew her," he says. I ignore the officers. We leave the street, and I tell Mohamed what happened. "*Kuntī khā'yfa?* Were you scared?" he asks. I tell him I was a little scared. "I understand," he says.

Mohamed hails a tuktuk, and we are soon on our way through the small streets of downtown Cairo. I ask Mohamed about his younger brother who was recently enrolled in the military and assigned a particularly vulnerable post in Sinai often targeted in drive-by shootings and bombings by militia groups in the area.

"He is okay," he responds. "We are keeping his post a secret from our mother, so please don't mention it. Because of her diabetes," he adds.

We soon arrive at his mother's apartment on the outskirts of Imbaba, and she quickly serves us a cup of tea. She asks me how much sugar I take; I tell her one teaspoon, but she gives me two. I ask about her diabetes. She tells me that she got it when her husband, Mohamed's father, passed away. "*Min il-za'l*, from the sadness," she says. "Because I loved him so much," she adds. Mohamed and his sister are sitting on the opposite bed, Mohamed's sister nods in agreement. Mohamed's mother tells me that she often worries that her blood sugar is not "*maṣbūṭ*, precise." She tells me that she once saw a neighbor cramp and die in the streets from his diabetes. "So, I only eat good things," she says, "like red chicken and bread and potatoes, but no rice." I smile back at her.

Mohamed abruptly changes the topic, "You know my real name is actually not Mohamed," he says. I first look at Mohamed, then at his mother and sister for confirmation. "Yes, it's true," Mohamed's mother nods and laughs. I look back at Mohamed. "My real name is Osama," he says. Mohamed gets his national identification card out of his pocket. "Look ..." He points to his name, written in Arabic, "Osama Mustafa." Mohamed's mother explains, "Mohamed's father wanted to name him Osama, but I wanted him to be Mohamed, so people would call me *Umm Mohamed*, mother of Mohamed. I told everyone to call him Mohamed instead of Osama, so with the government, *fī il-ḥukūma*, he is Osama, but everyone around here calls him Mohamed." We laugh at the story and I acknowledge Mohamed's mother for her wit.

Mohamed suggests we leave his mother to rest, "because of her diabetes," he explains. I nod and we get up to leave. Out of the building, Mohamed theatrically inhales and exhales slowly. "Finally," he exclaims, quickly adding, "Let's get out of here!" He hails a tuktuk, and we are soon once again on our way through the small streets of downtown Cairo. I observe the streets as we go. After a while, I ask Mohamed if he ever misses his old neighborhood. "Sometimes," he says, "but I don't miss all the *drama* of living with my family." He uses the English word for "drama." I smile, and we sit in silence for a while. He hesitates, and then asks, "You know the Arabic word *ḍaghṭ*, right?"

Summary

I end this chapter with Mohamed's story for several reasons. First, the story aims to remind the reader of the uncertainties, for example, of the political situation in Cairo that ran through most spheres of everyday life and the pressures this put on the lives of individuals moving through the city. Surely, Cairenes were better than I at moving safely through the streets of Cairo (they knew better than I not to idle in front of an office building for example) – but they did often recount similar experiences of uncertainty in relation to, for example, the security police. Upon telling an acquaintance about the above incident at the office building, he noted, "I feel like the streets in Egypt are for movement only. If you stop, someone will ask you why and who you are."

Another reason for drawing on the above ethnographic encounter is to illustrate the ways in which Mohamed, Mai, Reem, Maha, and others performed different acts of care for their elderly family members with the one aim of relieving them of experiences of *ḍaghṭ* that could potentially worsen their condition of type-2 diabetes. In Mohamed's case, this meant, for example, keeping his mother out of the loop of his younger brother's actual posting as a conscript in an attempt to shield his mother from the stress of constantly worrying about the lack of safety of this particular posting. Type-2 diabetes treatment within the families that I was working with in Cairo, in other words, revolved primarily around acts of care carried out by others within the family with the one purpose of relieving loved ones diagnosed with type-2 diabetes from physical and emotional strain.

Finally, by drawing on this closing story of Mohamed I wish to end the chapter by summing up its main argument – that relieving loved ones of experiences of *ḍaghṭ* did not simply make this *ḍaghṭ* go away. Rather, it shifted it to other family members who were left dealing with their own experiences of *ḍaghṭ*. The metabolism of individuals, in other words, merged into a metabolism of the common body of the family; the movements of one greatly affecting the movements of others. Type-2 diabetes in Cairo thus came to transmit not only, for example, by way of economic inflation, the climate, or concerns over polluted food and pharmaceutical drugs, but also through acts of care within the family household.

Note

1 Original song "Tab wana mali" first performed by Algerian singer Warda Al-Jazairia in 1973.

References

Al-Mohammad, Hayder. 2010. Towards an Ethics of Being-With: Intertwinements of Life in Post-Invasion Basra. *Ethnos* 75(4): 425–446.

Al-Mohammad, Hayder. 2012. A Kidnapping in Basra: The Struggles and Precariousness of Life in Postinvasion Iraq. *Cultural Anthropology* 27(4): 597–614.

Christensen, Fie Lund Lindegaard, and Jens Seeberg. 2017. Configuring the Autism Epidemic: Why Are So Few Girls Diagnosed? *Tidsskrift for Forskning i Sygdom Og Samfund* 26: 127–144.

Ghannam, Farha. 2013. *Live and Die Like a Man: Gender Dynamics in Urban Egypt*. Stanford University Press.

Grøn, Lone. 2017. Slægt, Hygge, Tid Og Sted: Familieperspektiver På Overvægtsepidemien. *Tidsskrift for Forskning i Sygdom Og Samfund* 26: 17–40.

Hamdy, Sherine F. 2012. *Our Bodies Belong to God: Organ Transplants, Islam, and the Struggle for Human Dignity in Egypt*. University of California Press.

Kleinman, Arthur. 2009. Caregiving: The Odyssey of Becoming More Human. *The Lancet* 373(9660): 292–293.

Mattingly, Cheryl, Lone Grøn, and Lotte Meinert. 2011. Chronic Homework in Emerging Borderlands of Healthcare. *Culture, Medicine, and Psychiatry* 35(3): 347–375.

Mol, Annemarie. 2008. *The Logic of Care: Health and the Problem of Patient Choice*. Routledge.
Moran-Thomas, Amy. 2019a. *Traveling with Sugar: Chronicles of a Global Epidemic*. University of California Press.
Moran-Thomas, Amy. 2019b. What Is Communicable? Unaccounted Injuries and "Catching" Diabetes in an Illegible Epidemic. *Cultural Anthropology* 34(4): 471–502.
Nielsen, Jeanette Lykkegård. 2017. Alkohol Og Relationalitet: Social Smitte Som Animistisk Fænomen i Sibirien. *Tidsskrift for Forskning i Sygdom Og Samfund* 26: 109–126.
Schielke, Samuli J. 2009. Being Good in Ramadan: Ambivalence, Fragmentation, and the Moral Self in the Lives of Young Egyptians. *The Journal of the Royal Anthropological Institute* 15: S24–S40.
Schielke, Samuli J. 2015. *Egypt in the Future Tense: Hope, Frustration, and Ambivalence before and after 2011*. Indiana University Press.
Seeberg, Jens, and Lotte Meinert. 2015. Can Epidemics Be Noncommunicable? Reflections on the Spread of "Noncommunicable" Diseases. *Medicine Anthropology Theory* 2(2): 54–71.

6 Novo

Mā huwa maraḍ il-sukkar? ("What is diabetes?") was written on the front page of a brochure produced and distributed across Cairo by Novo Nordisk during the time of my research in the years of 2015–2017. The brochure provided the reader with a firm answer to this question as well: obesity leads to type-2 diabetes, and potentially complicates all types of diabetes. As should be evident by now, this understanding of the primary cause of type-2 diabetes was promoted also by doctors and other healthcare personnel in Cairo; however, those diagnosed with type-2 diabetes themselves persistently questioned this etiology of "diabesity" and the treatment it promoted.

Sociologist Michel Foucault first argued in the late 1970s that modern forms of political thought and action are based on a certain kind of mentality that utilizes specific mechanisms in an attempt to align personal conduct with socio-political objectives. These mechanisms, he argued, include ways of calculation, technologies, discourses, and institutional setups (Foucault 1991). Social theorists Peter Miller and Nikolas Rose have summed up these ideas by Foucault as follows:

> To the extent that authoritative norms, calculative technologies and forms of evaluation can be translated into the values, decisions and judgements of citizens in their professional and personal capacities, they can function as part of the "self-steering" mechanisms of individuals. Hence, "free" individuals and "private" spaces can be "ruled" without breaching their formal autonomy.
>
> (Miller and Rose 2008:42)

DOI: 10.4324/9781003327684-6

Put differently, individuals may be affected, for example, through institutional setups and calculative technologies to act in specific ways, yet in the experience of those individuals, their actions are based entirely on their own free will. Foucault fittingly coined this mentality promoted by modern forms of political thought and action as "governmentality" (Foucault 1991).

In the first parts of this chapter, I draw on these theories by Foucault and others when arguing that Novo Nordisk attempted to appropriate certain mechanisms (such as institutional setups, specific policies, and the requirement to see certain documentation) in an attempt to make patients (or customers) and doctors in Cairo conform to specific ideas of what constitutes proper diabetes care. "We have to alter what they think," one Egyptian Novo employee argues later in this chapter, "We" being Novo Nordisk, and "they" being Egyptians with type-2 diabetes. Specifically, I illustrate how Novo Nordisk worked to enforce medical prescriptions commonly not used in Egypt, and how they facilitated practices of documentation in public clinics that were not required normally to document patient consultations. Through these points of analysis, I explore how Novo Nordisk appropriated specific understandings of certainty and objectivity in relation to diabetes care that contrary to its intentions carried the risk of generating uncertainties within their customers, for example, in relation to their course of treatment and the supply and distribution of medicine and medical technologies.

In the second part of the chapter, I attempt to gather together the arguments of the book; the ways in which uncertainties, *ḍaghṭ*, and type-2 diabetes intertwined with etiologies of "diabesity," multinational pharmaceutical companies and international guidelines throughout my research in Cairo. By drawing on an empirical encounter from an outpatient clinic for people with diabetes in Aarhus, Denmark – linked by way of Novo Nordisk to the outpatient clinic I had worked with in Cairo the most – I wish to finally discuss the ways in which such intertwinements carried the risk of undermining individuals and their personal experiences and struggles of living with type-2 diabetes in Egypt.

I first turn to a Novo Care Center situated in the middle-class neighborhood of Dokki in Cairo; a clinic owned and run by Novo Nordisk with the main purpose of distributing the NovoPen (a device used to inject insulin), as well as educating people diagnosed with all types of diabetes about their condition. Here I spent time with Aaliyah and Nadia, two pharmacists employed by Novo Nordisk to instruct customers in the proper use of the NovoPen and to teach them about diabetes in general.

The Novo Care Center (September 2015)

Eight women are gathered around the desk. Aaliyah, the pharmacist, is trying to get their attention. The women are all speaking in loud voices, advising one another on what to eat and not to eat, what to cook and not to cook for their husbands. One of the women suddenly takes off one of her shoes, places her bare foot on the desk, and points to her toes and sides of her foot. She starts explaining that it's important for the other women to check their husbands' feet for ulcers. Aaliyah nods as she quiets down the group, and asks them to focus on "*il-'alam*, the pen." The office feels cool from the air-conditioner. The place is clean and neat with new furniture and TV screens on the walls, airing the same handful of informational slides on diabetes. The Novo Nordisk logo is placed in the bottom-right corner of the slides.

Aaliyah is giving the women instructions on how to use the NovoPen; how to put the insulin inside, how to adjust the dosage, where to inject the insulin, how to store the insulin, and how to change the needle after every injection. "You mean once a month?" one of the women interrupts. "No ..." Aaliyah declares, "After every injection you should change the needle." The women all start arguing. "Once a week?" "Every other day?" Aaliyah finally relents that if the women's husbands insist on reusing the needle, they should only reuse it a maximum of three times. "*Da il-ʾakbar*, that's the maximum," she says in a strict tone. Aaliyah adds that if the needle is bent in any way, it should not be reused at all.

Aaliyah finally gives the women some dietary advice, handing out brochures of foods considered good and not good for someone with diabetes. "These foods are not good," she says, and points to one of the many lists in the brochure, "for example, mangos and dates." The women burst out laughing. One jokingly says, "I think I have to go home and empty the fridge."

Nadia, the other pharmacist, is sitting next to me. I lean over and ask her about the disposable needles. She quietly tells me that one needle costs about two Egyptian pounds, "And most inject twice a day, so ..."[1]

Two other women enter the center. Nadia greets them and invites them to follow her further into the office. I tag along as well. One of the women inquiries about an insulin pen for her husband. "His doctor told him to get it from here, I bought the insulin already." She hands Nadia a bag of insulin. Nadia glances into the bag, nods, and then asks about "*il-prescription*." The woman shakes her head, indicating that she doesn't understand what Nadia means by *il-prescription*. Nadia explains, "I need a paper from your husband's doctor stating that he needs the pen." Nadia adds that she cannot give the women the pen before she sees the paper.

The women start arguing with Nadia. "I can get the pen today, and return tomorrow with *il-wara'a*, the paper," one of the women says. Nadia says no. The women insist. Nadia says no again, "I can't." She finally says, "*Il-company* needs the paper." Nadia points to a big white and blue sign hanging on the wall illuminating the logo and name of Novo Nordisk. The women thank Nadia and leave the center.

Aaliyah has joined us in the back office. The other women have left with the NovoPens and instructions for their husbands. A woman enters the office, and walks determinedly toward us. "If I had two sandwiches for breakfast, what should I eat now?" she asks without greeting us. It's approximately 11:30am. I recognize the woman from earlier in the day. Aaliyah clarifies some of the woman's questions, and the woman quickly leaves the center again. Aaliyah explains that the woman did not actually have a prescription for the NovoPen herself, but her father did, and he recently passed away. The woman is now using her father's pen instead of a regular syringe to inject her insulin. "She is going to use the pen no matter what I say, so I might as well give her instructions," Aaliyah explains.

There is a steady flow of patients coming in and out of the center. One woman enters with her young daughter, she is approximately 8 years old. The daughter has just been diagnosed with diabetes, and advised to use the NovoPen and insulin. Nadia asks for the prescription, and for the girl's birthdate. The girl's mother says she does not have a prescription, and she does not remember the girl's birthdate. "She was born on a Friday," she says. Nadia says that they need to return with the exact birthdate and the prescription. The girl asks to use the toilet before leaving. She passes the water dispenser and drinks three cups of water before using the toilet. Nadia glances at the girl, and then turns to the girl's mother, "You need to come back with the prescription immediately, your daughter clearly needs the insulin."

Principles ("*Il-Company* Needs the Paper")

At the time of the above empirical encounter in 2015, Novo Nordisk had approximately 30 of the above-portrayed Novo Care Centers spread across Egypt. A large portion of these centers were located adjacent to privately owned pharmacies, others were independent centers. On a good day, I was told, the centers would be consulted by about 300 people altogether. The center portrayed above was the largest one in Egypt in terms of number of patient consultations per day. It was situated in the heart of Dokki, a middle-class neighborhood in Cairo, though it served people from all over the city and from many different segments of society. The main purpose of the Novo Care Centers was to distribute the Novo insulin pen (NovoPen) to customers. This included teaching people how to use the pen properly, as well as teaching them about diabetes more generally (common dietary advice, symptoms of late complications, how to treat acute cases of hypoglycemia, low blood sugar, and so on).

The centers also had the role of filing reports to the head office in Denmark in cases of dysfunctional pens or in other "unusual" cases, in the words of the manager of the center, for example, if patients had suffered allergic reactions while using the NovoPen (and insulin). In the words of Aaliyah (portrayed above), the role of the Novo Care Center was to mold people's habits and thoughts in relation to diabetes. "We have to alter what they think," she summed up her work in the center.

Most of the staff at the Novo Care Center in Dokki held master's degrees in pharmaceuticals, biology, or similar fields from private, highly esteemed universities across Cairo. All belonged to the upper class, spoke English fluently, and lived either in the upscale neighborhood of Zamalek close to Dokki, or in one of the gated communities (or "compounds") just outside Cairo.

The consultations at the Novo Care Center differed from those, for example, at the public medical clinic in Giza (portrayed in Chapter 2 and later in this chapter as well), as Nadia, Aaliyah, and others in the center were focusing on patient education, rather than specific blood sugar measurements, adjustments of medicine, and so on. Still, the consultations at the Novo Care Center were similar to those at the doctoral clinics in terms of the arguments and discussions between patients (or customers) and healthcare personnel. This is evident in the above encounter where, for example, the group of women were all objecting to the notion of discarding the disposable needles when they had been used only once, and in their laughter at Aaliyah's suggestion not to eat mangos and dates when diagnosed with diabetes.

As mentioned in the above, the main purpose of the Novo Care Centers was to distribute the NovoPen, a device used to inject insulin. The NovoPen is used as a replacement for the common syringe. The pen has many advantages as compared to a syringe in relation to usability, precision, portability, and hygiene. In Cairo, those who had switched from syringes to the pen pointed also to the fact that the injecting of insulin hurts much less when using a pen compared to a common syringe. The NovoPen needs to be filled, of course, with insulin. In Novo's terms, this insulin goes by the name of Penfill. In order to get access to the NovoPen at the above Novo Care Centers, people had to show a prescription from their doctor stating that he/she advised the patient to use the NovoPen and insulin specifically.

As mentioned in Chapter 2, Egyptians do not usually need a prescription to access most medicine or medical technologies. The need to show a prescription to access the NovoPen was thus not a need established by Egyptian law, but rather one held by Novo Nordisk ("*Il-company* needs the paper," as Nadia expressed it above). As illustrated throughout the above encounter, several people were turned away daily from the Novo Care Center in Dokki because they did not have such a formal prescription from their doctor. According to Nadia and Aaliyah, many would argue with them before leaving the center, and return another day with "*il-wara'a*, the paper." During the time that I spent in the center, this was my experience as well. Many of those who were told to return to the doctor to retrieve a prescription would respond with something along the lines of, "I just came from the doctor, he told me to come here!" In short, neither doctors nor patients (or customers) appeared to fully understand the importance of having a prescription to show to the employees at the center. In fact, doctors would frequently call the center confused as to what was required of them.

Egyptian Novo employees, in contrast, understood the notion of a prescription in a legal sense, but they were also aware that most of the people consulting the center were not familiar with this specific idea. This ability to understand the perspectives of both Novo and their customers provided Egyptian Novo employees with a unique expertise, but it also left them with great frustration. In fact, Nadia and Aaliyah had used that exact English word, "frustrating," when outlining how they had to reject (often sick) people because they did not have the right papers from their doctor. Nadia explicitly expressed the difficulties of turning away the young girl portrayed above, and her concern as to whether or not the girl's mother would ever return with a prescription or if she might decide on a different treatment altogether (or none at all). "She [the mother] made the effort to come here, perhaps this was not easy, and then I had to turn her away because she did not have the papers we need … whereas her daughter clearly needed the insulin," Nadia told me.

Let me be clear on the notion of prescriptions in Egypt: doctors prescribe medicine in the sense that they advise their patients on what medicine to take (and this they do extensively). Doctors scribble down names of drugs on sticky notes, snippets of paper, napkins, and so on, and hand them out to patients during most consultations – but these papers are not official papers with stamps and signatures that have a legal status without which patients cannot retrieve their medicine from the pharmacy. As a result, prescribing medicine in Egypt can be considered to be mostly a social act, rather than a legal one (though there are a few pharmaceuticals such as certain opioids and psychopharmaceuticals that do require legal prescriptions, and that can only be retrieved from a few pharmacies in Cairo and the country at large). Anthropologists Sjaak van der Geest, Anita Hardon, and Susan Whyte argue on the social act of prescribing medicine, "It demonstrates the physician's concern. Through prescriptions, doctors show their patients that they recognize their complaints and are trying to help them" (Geest, Hardon, and Whyte 1996:160). The type of prescription enforced in the Novo Care Centers were prescriptions in a legal sense, and less so in a social sense. In other words, in Novo's perspective, prescriptions were supposed to be vested with authority, validity, and certainty in ways that prescriptions (on napkins and sticky notes) are commonly not in Egypt.

According to Nadia, Aaliyah, and others working with Novo Nordisk in Egypt, the "need" of "*il-company*" to see such a legal piece of paper was related to specific ideas about the proper handling of pharmaceuticals (and in this case also the proper handling of medical technologies). I heard Novo employees discuss the "responsibility" taken on by the company when enforcing prescriptions in a legal sense in an attempt to "control" the use of pharmaceuticals, to prevent "overprescribing" (on napkins and sticky notes) and "self-prescribing" (people who were making their own decisions about what medicine to take and who were able to retrieve them from any pharmacy without a prescription in a legal sense). Novo clearly promoted the idea that access to medicine (and medical technologies) should be based not on free will, but rather on a redistribution of such decisions to so-called experts (in this case to doctors). Novo thus enforced the use of prescriptions in a legal sense as a "technical device," to borrow a term from Miller and Rose, rendering it possible to not only represent certain objectives, but also to intervene and act upon individuals (Miller and Rose 2008:30–2).

Whereas Miller and Rose have outlined Foucault's term of "governmentality" as capturing the ability to govern "at a distance"

(Miller and Rose 2008:26), the enforcement of the use of legal prescriptions in the Novo Care Centers rather appeared to be a very direct and evident way of governing (or attempting to govern). This is evident in the specific objections of the women in the above encounter ("I can get the pen today, and return tomorrow with *il-wara'a*, the paper"), but it was also evident in many similar arguments and objections throughout my time in the center. In summary, the attempt by Novo Nordisk to promote specific medical ethics in relation to the handling of medicine and medical technologies in Egypt seemed, first and foremost, to generate confusion and uncertainty among those diagnosed with type-2 diabetes who frequented the Novo Care Center in Dokki – as opposed to generate certainty in the workings of both the company and its products.

In general, Novo was vesting documents with an authority and legal status that was rarely acknowledged or honored, for example, by the authorities in Egypt. Political scientist Timothy Mitchell has outlined how European colonial rule in Egypt and elsewhere attempted to transform local administrative systems from systems characterized largely by "arbitrariness" to systems characterized by so-called "universalism" and consistency. He writes, "In non-European government the exceptional was the rule; power gained its strength from its arbitrariness. Modern government, like modern science, the European believed, was based upon principles true in every country. Its strength lay in its universalism" (Mitchell 2002:54). Mitchell elaborates specifically in relation to British rule in Egypt, "The political economy of Egypt was to be reestablished on the basis of principles true in every country" (Mitchell 2002:55). Mitchell outlines how this process also entailed the vesting of legal papers and documents with an unprecedented authority.

To this day, papers, documents, stamps, and signatures are intrinsic to Egyptian bureaucracy (as it is, I suspect, in most places), but so is the notion coined by Mitchell, or the British colonial rule, of "arbitrariness" – the sense that papers can always be torn apart, deemed not necessary, not sufficient or counterfeit by people working within the system. In other words, papers and documents only carry authority and a legal status as long as people choose to uphold this authority and status. As argued throughout this book, power is maintained by the Egyptian state precisely by generating such uncertainties. However, these mechanisms of uncertainty greatly contrasted with the ways in which Novo Nordisk appropriated ideas of "universalism" and certainty, evident, for example, in the attempts to introduce legal medical prescriptions in an

Egyptian context, but also in the ways they engaged with Egyptian authorities and bureaucracy more generally.

During my fieldwork in Cairo in 2015, I learned that Novo Nordisk had signed an agreement with the Egyptian Ministry of Health to offer 6,000 NovoPens for free per year. In turn, the Ministry of Health had to buy 700,000 packs of Penfill (to be given to Egyptian patients for free or released on the market at a subsidized rate). The Egyptian government would thus save money from not having to purchase the pens, but with this money, they should purchase Penfill (insulin from Novo Nordisk). In the words of a Novo employee, "They are saving this money to buy better treatment, better medications for the patient." (Several Novo employees hinted that locally produced insulin was "not really effective"; in fact, it was "like water.")

However, the Egyptian Ministry of Health did not meet their side of the agreement. In the words of the Novo employee cited above, "When we came to the implementation phase of this project, this was not really quite easy to implement. They [The Ministry of Health] said ... okay ... you give us the free NovoPens and then we will see whether or not we will buy the Penfills." In other words, a written contract between Novo Nordisk and The Egyptian Ministry of Health was viewed quite differently by the two parties. Novo for one (initially anyways) seemed to view the contract as certain and final, and the breaking of the contract as illegal. The Egyptian Ministry of Health seemed to view the contract as vested with little certainty and authority.

The Diabetes Clinic in Giza (September 2015)

Karim holds his iPhone in one hand, and steers the car with the other. He is looking intensely at the GPS on his phone. "Sorry, I don't know this area of Cairo very well," he says. I lean back into my seat, enjoying the cool air inside of the car, and Cairo passing by on the outside.

"So, I can't believe you usually take the metro," Karim laughs. "I only ever took it once, and I grew up in Cairo!" We both laugh. "Well, it's easy and cheap," I say. I look over at Karim; he is wearing a suit, and is looking at the street in front of us through an expensive pair of sunglasses. His Novo Nordisk employee card hangs on a blue lanyard around his neck. "So, about the clinic ..." he says.

We are on our way to the diabetes clinic in Giza, the one financed partially by Novo, but run by the public hospital where it is located. Karim's position at Novo Nordisk is to manage the relationship between the company and the clinic. "Our biggest challenge is the staff ..." Karim pauses for a while. "It's some kind of an MOH [Ministry of Health] problem that doctors do not really work fulltime even though they are paid to work fulltime. It's not exactly quite clear ... what's definitely certain is that all governmental institutions here in Egypt, they have a similar problem with workers."

I adjust my phone to make sure it is still recording – Karim suggested to make the most of our time in the car and invited me to record our conversation. He continues, "This has something to do with the salaries they are getting paid. Of course, they realize that it's not worth coming to the hospital if they get paid much more in a private hospital or if they have their own clinic. So, officially, on paper, they are hired by this hospital full-time, but unofficially, the personnel rarely show up." Karim drives through the gates to the hospital, greeting the security guard as we pass him. He parks the car in front of the clinic.

The clinic itself is shiny and bright on the inside; a stark contrast to the rest of the hospital. Karim glances at me, recognizing my thoughts before I speak – "Yeah, everything here is very white," he says. We both laugh.

Karim tells me to sit with one of the senior doctors, Rania, for a couple of sessions. He needs to talk to the director of the hospital, and then he will give me a grand tour of the clinic. He knocks on the door to one of the consultation rooms, interrupting a session with a patient. Rania, the doctor happily greets me, gesturing for me to take a seat next to her. Karim closes the door behind him.

Rania turns to look at Fatima, the patient, who is sitting in front of her. Fatima is in her 40s, and has recently been diagnosed with type-2 diabetes. "There is no reason for us to fight," Rania says, addressing Fatima. Rania adds, "You have to know what you can eat and what is forbidden." Fatima starts arguing. She is shouting in a loud and shrill voice.

The air-conditioning is humming in the background, keeping the Cairo summer heat at bay. Rania sighs and opens Fatima's file on the computer. She starts ticking off several symptoms without asking Fatima about the symptoms. "Weight gain. Fatigue. Excessive thirst." Fatima is still arguing, commenting that her blood sugars are high because she is "upset" and "sad," not because she is not eating correctly. Rania doesn't respond, but keeps checking off symptoms in Fatima's file.

A nurse opens the door and walks across the consultation room. She is drinking a Coke, straight out of the shiny red can. She picks up a stethoscope, and quickly leaves the room without speaking a word. A patient abruptly opens the door and walks in. Rania tells her to leave immediately. Rania closes Fatima's file on the computer, and tells Fatima to go lie down on the examination bed. Rania slowly gets up from behind her desk to examine her. On her way to the examination bed she tells me in English, "Bad habits … one of the main causes of wrong treatment. Write that down …" She points to my notebook. Rania quietly examines Fatima before suddenly exclaiming in Arabic, so Fatima understands, "She claims her measurements are too high because she is sad. But that is wrong!"

There is a lot of noise coming from the waiting room. People seem to be shouting at each other, and a nurse screams at someone to "calm down!" Rania abruptly opens the door, quickly scanning everyone in the waiting room. She doesn't speak a word, but a hush falls over the waiting room as everyone turns to look at her. Rania leaves the door open, and returns to the desk. Fatima leaves the consultation room, and Nadwa, another woman in her 40s with type-2 diabetes, shuts the door behind her as she enters.

Nadwa hands Rania a piece of paper with her lab results. Rania looks at Nadwa's results; her blood sugar is rather high, but Nadwa seems happy. "It is lower than last time," Nadwa says.

Rania looks at Nadwa, "They are lower?" She promptly adds, "You need to eat healthier." She scans the lab results once again, and points to some other measurements, "and drink more water," she says.

Nadwa says, "But I have a lot of water in my body …"

"That's why you need to drink a lot of water," Rania says without elaborating further. "You need to learn what to eat and what not to eat." Nadwa simply smiles at Rania and me. Rania looks at her, "Why are you so happy?" she asks. "You have had diabetes for 15 years and it still looks this bad!" Rania looks at me as if she is about to give up. She points to Nadwa, and then to Nadwa's lab results. Rania says to me in English, "This is a suicide attempt."

Nadwa is looking at both of us, still smiling, shifting nervously back and forth in her seat. I wonder if she understands the English.

Rania opens the checklist of symptoms on the computer to be saved electronically to Nadwa's file. She starts ticking off symptoms without asking Nadwa. She reads aloud from the checklist,

"Weight gain? ... *of course* ..." as she checks off "weight gain" in the system.[2]

(Non-)Compliance

During my fieldwork in Cairo in 2015, Novo Nordisk was collaborating with the Egyptian Ministry of Health to renovate 26 public outpatient clinics for people with diabetes across the country. The one in Giza was the first of these clinics to open. The details of the collaboration meant that Novo would finance extensive renovations and state-of-the-art equipment to be used in the clinics, but the clinics would be run by the hospitals (and thus ultimately by the state). Novo was to finance the fixed expenses, and, in turn, the hospital would cover the running expenses (such as salaries, disposable kits, gloves, and so on).

The clinic in Giza was organized so that patients would, first, see a nurse for basic checkups and vitals (for example, weight and blood pressure). Next, they would see an endocrinologist, who would assess their lab results and vitals, check their legs and feet for ulcers, and outline a proper course of medical treatment. If relevant, the endocrinologist would refer the patient to the ophthalmologist (eye specialist), cardiologist (heart specialist), nephrologist (kidney specialist), dietician, and/or specialist in diabetic foot ulcers. All specialties were available in the clinic with consultation rooms next to the endocrinologist. In fact, one of the primary aims of the clinic was to gather all relevant specialists within the same clinic for easy access and timely treatment.

The clinic also ran its own pharmacy and electronic medicine handling system. An important point to emphasize here is the fact that doctors could prescribe medicine as they saw fit. Hence, there were no expectations to prioritize Novo's products as such. In fact, during my 2015 fieldwork, Novo had recently lost a public procurement to another medical company, and thus Penfill, for example, was not available at the pharmacy in the clinic. In summary, the clinic was considered to be a free public clinic, albeit a bright and shiny one.

In reality, however, the clinic did not work as intended. As reflected in the above conversation with Karim, who managed the relation between Novo and the hospital, the above-mentioned specialists were rarely available in the clinic (at least not as frequently as they were supposed to be). The pharmacy also suffered from a lack of medicine due to the frequent shortages across the country. Furthermore, some medical companies downright refused to do business with the hospital, as the hospital, apparently, had a poor history of paying their bills. In addition, the hospital did not cover most of the running expenses they had agreed to initially, which left the clinic in chronic need of, for example, hygienic supplies such as disposable gloves and bedding, disposable kits used to operate machines, and so on. Furthermore, Karim pointed to the lack of cleaning in the clinic as an issue, "They are cleaning it, but not regularly. They are cleaning it, but not according to international standards." In Karim's opinion, this was clearly not good enough. He summed up Novo's cooperation with the clinic as follows, "When we started this project it was a partnership; 'we [Novo] get you the hard stuff, and you [the hospital] get the easy stuff.' But when we went through with the project, they didn't really want to get even the easy things."

The main reason the hospital did not cover these "easy things" was, of course, not a lack of willingness, but rather the fact that the hospital was greatly underfunded by the Ministry of Health (which in turn was greatly underfunded). Although Novo Nordisk had secured a specific institutional setup for the clinic on paper, as well as certain standards of care in an attempt to improve diabetes care in the area (and eventually across the country at large), they were, once again, faced with the fact that contracts entered into with the Egyptian Ministry of Health were not necessarily vested with much certainty and authority.

Medical literature often discusses the level of "compliance" in a patient, using the phrasing that compliance is "high" or "low" in an individual patient or within a group of patients with specific characteristics (see, for example, Cramer et al. 2008 for a literature review on the "significance of compliance" in the treatment of diabetes). "Compliance" refers to the degree to which a patient is likely to follow professional instructions in relation to treatment, such as, for example, medical and dietary advice. Whereas I never heard Egyptian doctors use the term "compliant" or "non-compliant" in relation to a patient, I heard many Egyptian Novo employees use the English word "compliance" directly in relation to customers, as well as when explaining the workings of others such as the Ministry of Health and Egyptian healthcare personnel (including doctors). In the perspective of Karim and others at Novo Nordisk, the hospital director, for example, was "non-compliant" in supplying the clinic with running expenses and with proper cleaning; doctors were "non-compliant" with regard to their working hours; and the Ministry of Health was generally "non-compliant" regarding most agreements, even those that were written in a contract.

In many ways, the term "compliance" (and the antonym of "non-compliance") reflects back to Foucault's notion of "governmentality" in its reference to the ability or non-ability of patients (and others) to self-regulate according to specific objectives (for example, in relation to specific ideas of what constitutes proper diabetes care). As mentioned previously, Miller and Rose have argued that the appropriation of certain "technologies" (such as institutional setups), "seeks to act upon and instrumentalize the self-regulating propensities of individuals in order to ally them with socio-political objectives" (Miller and Rose 2008:51). In the case of the clinic in Giza, Novo was clearly using the institutional setup, facilities, and agreements to affect both patients and staff in certain ways. Only, the "technologies" of Novo Nordisk were not sufficient to bring about the desired effects – rather, the company was left with an apparent "non-compliant" medical staff and with "non-compliant" authorities.

One of the outcomes of the collaboration between Novo Nordisk and public clinics across the country was the ability to build a national electronic database or registry of Egyptians diagnosed with diabetes. The database was supposed to be linked to the National Institute of Diabetes and Endocrinology, which is a part of the Egyptian Ministry of Health. According to the contract, Novo would be granted access to this data in return for renovating and providing public diabetes clinics across Egypt with state-of-the-art equipment. Karim explained the purpose of the database: "For the first time we can actually get a glimpse of how many diabetics we have in Egypt. Of course, that means that they have to go to these specific clinics, otherwise we don't have an accurate number, but it will be a great sample. It will also be a way to know how they are treated and not treated." In other words, Novo would ideally be able to use the data to research and promote certain products, and the Ministry of Health would be able to gather an unprecedented national database of a broad range of general public health information.

During my research at the clinic in 2015, the final stages of this project were yet to be actualized, as the Ministry of Health, once again, did not honor their side of the contract. According to Karim, this had little to do with the fact that the ministry did not want to share the patient data. Rather, it had to do with a lack of public funding, and thus the inability to get the technology up and running properly. However, from other examples of the Egyptian authorities not honoring their contracts with Novo Nordisk, I suspect that it might also have something to do with the leverage maintained by the Egyptian Ministry of Health in their relation to Novo Nordisk by withholding the data. Either way, Novo Nordisk had financed the renovation of the public clinic in Giza, including providing computers and software to be used during consultations, but the data had yet to be gathered centrally and released to the company.

It also became evident during my observations that doctors would often tick off patient symptoms in the software based solely on their own assessments (for example, if a patient showed a particularly elevated blood sugar level, the doctor would often tick off "Weight gain" automatically without actually knowing if the person had gained weight over the last couple of months). Other symptoms asked for by the software were left completely out of the conversation between the doctor and the patient, and were thus never ticked off as a problem. These included "Impotence" and "Loss of / decrease in libido." As illustrated in Chapter 2, diabetes consultations often followed two different lines of arguments and discussions altogether; whereas patients focused primarily on experiences of *ḍaghṭ*, pressure, including specific situations that had "upset" them or made them feel particularly "sad," as with Fatima in the above example, the doctors would rather follow a line of questions related to the etiology of "diabesity." Furthermore, the clinic in Giza was preoccupied with clarifying a list of symptoms in relation to the patients provided by Novo Nordisk such as "weight gain," "excessive thirst," "urination," "fatigue," "numbness," and "diarrhea."

From a Novo perspective, doctors were compliant in the sense that they were typing in data for every patient in the clinic. However, in my observations, the reported data rarely corresponded with symptoms actually voiced by the patients or with actual physiological measurements. Rather, Rania and others appeared to use the software system primarily to exemplify and emphasize poor treatment and self-care in their communication with patients ("Weight gain? ... *of course* ..." Rania noted in the above). Rania and other healthcare providers, in other words, made use of the software provided by Novo Nordisk, but they used it in ways that I suspect were not entirely intended by the company.

Dewey outlined in 1929 how the Latin word "data" originally means "givens," but that it would be more fitting to think of it as "takens." He argued, "*as* data they are *selected* from this total original subject-matter which gives the impetus to knowing; they are discriminated for a purpose: that, namely, of affording signs or evidence to define and locate a problem, and thus give a clew [*sic*] to its resolution" (Dewey 1929:178). Whyte similarly elaborates on these ideas of Dewey: "[the data is] discriminated and chosen for the purpose of locating and resolving a problem" (Whyte 1997:20). Novo had clearly chosen specific symptoms (and topics of interest) to build into the software used in the clinic in Giza, based on already defined notions of what constitutes the "problem" of diabetes as an overall disease category; sadness and stress, for example, were not included as part of this problem. Drawing once again on the notion of Miller and Rose, the software became a "technology" that affected the very structure and content of the consultations between patients and doctors, arguably with the intention to better qualify the consultations and overall treatment of the patients. However, as opposed to making room for the concerns of the patients, the consultations, I will argue, primarily made room for the concerns of Novo Nordisk. Once again, an attempt by Novo to appropriate certain medical ethics – in this case by implementing patient documentation and structuring the consultations in certain ways – caused uncertainties in regards to treatment and in relation to the healthcare personnel among the patients that frequented the clinic.

The above example of the software implemented in the public diabetes clinic in Giza speaks also to the ways in which knowledge or research is produced on a more general level: Which problems are emphasized and which are not? What data is "taken" and what is not? Who "takes" the data and what may be their agenda? Which solutions or treatments are subsequently promoted and which are not? In other words, the above example serves to remind us of the complexities of scientific thinking; intrinsic to that which becomes known about a given subject, there will be questions that were never raised and answers that were never picked up on. Anthropologist Amy Moran-Thomas fittingly argues from her work on diabetes in Belize: "data get lost when we assume in advance that we know what a condition's markers look like" (Moran-Thomas 2019:475).

During my time in the clinic, Karim never questioned the ways in which Rania and others were reporting data into the software provided by Novo. Some of the doctors working in the clinic in Giza (and in other future clinics across Egypt as well) had, as it turned out, been on a trip to an outpatient clinic for people with diabetes in Aarhus, Denmark, in order to learn how to properly (in the perspective of Novo Nordisk) conduct a diabetes consultation – including how to properly document consultations. This trip was paid for by Novo, and had taken place a short time before the clinic in Giza was opened in 2014. Novo, in other words, seemed to aim at Rania (who had actually not been on the trip to Denmark) and others to use the software portrayed in the above in ways that mirrored the workings of Danish doctors trained to legally document consultations as accurately as possible. Only, doctors in Egypt are not used to documenting medical consultations; in fact, in all of the clinics and hospitals that I visited in Egypt during my research, it was only the one clinic in Giza that displayed even a set of computers, and that clearly expected doctors to document each consultation meticulously – encouraged by Novo Nordisk. However, similar to the arguments of the previous parts of this chapter, the authority and certainty vested by Novo Nordisk – in this case in medical documentation – was not appropriated or implemented in such ways by the doctors in Giza.

Even though I did not have the opportunity to "follow" the data plotted into the files at the clinic by Rania and others (as Appadurai 1988 would follow the "thing"), and thus examine how the data was later utilized by Novo Nordisk (and the Egyptian Ministry of Health), the examples outlined above may still serve to cement questions raised at the beginning of this book, such as how facts come to be facts in the first place? Before turning to sum up on this question and others from the book, I will first turn to the diabetes clinic in Aarhus, Denmark, which staff from the above public clinic in Giza had visited in 2014.

The Diabetes Clinic in Aarhus (October 2017)

The nurse asks Anne how she is doing.

"I started working in a candy shop and I accidentally ate too much candy this weekend, I have to stop doing that," Anne says. Anne is 16 years old and has type-1 diabetes. She tells the nurse, "So please don't consider my blood sugars from this weekend, because they are really bad." The nurse smiles at Anne while attempting to find her blood sugars on the computer screen. Out of the blue, Anne asks the nurse if the hospital can stop sending their text messages to her mother's phone, and instead send them to her phone directly.

"It's a bit annoying that my mother gets all my messages when they are actually meant for me," she says. The nurse opens a different tab in Anne's file. She scans the screen for a cell-phone number. The nurse finds a number and reads it aloud. "Yeah, that's my mother's number," Anne says, as Anne's mother sits quietly next to her, but then interjects.

"I would still like to get the messages as well," Anne's mother says. She quickly looks at Anne and says, "Perhaps I check my phone more than you do?" Anne glares back at her.

"Seriously? I check my phone all the time!" Anne says. They both turn to look at the nurse.

"Can we both get the messages?" Anne's mother asks. The nurse explains that the system will only accept one cell-phone number.

"Type in mine!" Anne says. The nurse starts typing. Anne's mother turns to address Anne.

"Okay, but then you have to remember to tell me as well, so I can help you remember the time of your consultations," she says. Anne doesn't reply. She looks at me, smiling. I smile back at her. Anne's mother catches our smiles, and breaks a smile as well, squeezing Anne's hand.

The nurse is finally ready with the blood sugar measurements. She turns the screen toward Anne. Anne leans over to get a better view, and they study the various graphs and tables of blood sugar levels intensely. Anne speaks up before the nurse, pointing to some high blood sugar levels at night.

"I don't know if I need to consider my carbohydrates a bit more at night?" she asks. She looks at the nurse. Before the nurse gets to respond, Anne has another suggestion ready, "Or perhaps ..." They debate back and forth for a while, and I lean over to study the measurements as well. Anne's levels are indeed quite high around midnight.

"I was previously really scared that my blood sugar would drop too much while sleeping, maybe that's why I let it get a bit high at night. But the rest looks better regulated than it has been for years," Anne says.

"Your numbers aren't jumping up and down as much as before because your body is almost fully grown. There are fewer hormones in your body affecting your diabetes. Everything is sort of calming down," the nurse explains. Anne nods quietly, eyes still fixed on the screen.

"I think I have to refresh my knowledge of the carbohydrate rules," Anne says. The nurse asks Anne if she knows of the "carbohydrate app" by the Danish Diabetes Association. Anne picks up her phone and starts looking for the app.

The nurse turns to her and says, "Look ... It's okay to be careful at night. You shouldn't slam your blood sugar all the way down to 6 before you go to bed. But maybe you can adjust it just a little bit. If you lower the blood sugar too much at night, perhaps it will be too low in the morning. So, you are treading on a fine line. You have to adjust a little bit, but be careful while you do it."

Anne picks up her insulin pump and starts pressing some of the buttons. She chats with the nurse, and they agree on what exactly should be changed. Anne changes the settings herself and tucks the pump away.

"I completely trust the pump. I actually just do what it tells me to do," Anne comments.

"The pump is actually quite dumb when you think about it. It doesn't regulate well itself, you have to do that. It gives you suggestions, but that's all," the nurse says.

"Yes, it's true. It can't think at all. You have to think yourself," Anne's mother says. She looks at her daughter and then asks, "Do you think maybe you are more careful not to lower your blood sugar at night because you changed bedrooms and no longer sleep in the room next to me and dad?"

"No, that's not it at all ..." Anne says.

The nurse asks Anne to measure her current blood sugar level. Anne quickly gets a needle, testing strips, and a measuring device out of her purse. She gets up to wash her hands before measuring; she clearly knows the routine well. Anne's mother explains that she doesn't get too involved with Anne's diabetes anymore.

"Yeah, you don't really ask if I have measured my blood sugars and stuff like that," she says. "I know my diabetes better than anyone else anyways," she adds.

The nurse looks at Anne and then says, "You know, that is true, but it is very important, even as an adult, always to share the responsibility of your diabetes with someone else." Anne quietly nods while looking at her phone, checking up on the different diabetes apps she is now downloading.

"When she has been out drinking [alcohol], she always goes to sleep on the couch in the living room so that her father and I can measure her blood sugars in the morning, and wake her up if she needs some juice or something," Anne's mother reveals. We all laugh. Anne's mother adds, "In *that* case, it's still okay for us to help out."

The (Un)Certainty of Facts

The above consultation represents the majority of consultations that I observed at the diabetes clinic in Aarhus with patients diagnosed both with type-1 and type-2 diabetes. Compared to the clinic in Giza, there were many differences between the two settings. First and foremost, the general use of technologies among people with diabetes in Denmark was very high compared to people with diabetes (both type-1 and type-2 diabetes) in Egypt: smartphones, apps, insulin pens, pumps, and blood sugar measuring devices were everyday tools used by most people with diabetes at the clinic in Aarhus (and rarely used among people with neither type-1 nor type-2 diabetes who attended, for example, the clinic in Giza). Insulin pumps, for example, such as the one used by Anne in the above, were particularly common among young people with diabetes who frequented the clinic in Aarhus. In Cairo, the insulin pen (such as the NovoPen) appeared as the most recent technological advancement available.

None of the people that I knew in Cairo who were dependent on insulin had ever heard of an insulin pump. In short, the pump is placed on the body and injects insulin on a continuous basis throughout the day; the person using the pump does not have to remember to inject insulin at specific times, because the pump does that automatically. In addition, the pump measures the person's blood sugar levels frequently and stores this data for later analysis (mainly for consultations with health professionals). Based on these blood sugar measurements, the pump may suggest adjustments in the preset dosages of insulin (which the person using the pump may accept or reject).

At the Aarhus clinic, Anne placed a high level of trust in her insulin pump ("I actually just do what it tells me to do"). Both Anne's mother and the nurse subsequently warned Anne that the pump, in fact, was rather "dumb" ("It can't think at all," as Anne's mother put it). Contrary to most of the patients I observed across various medical consultations in Egypt, Anne had to be encouraged to question medical facts presented to her, in this case by her insulin pump. In general, there was very little questioning of medical advice during consultations in Aarhus compared to those that I had observed in Cairo, regardless of whether the advice was given by a doctor, a nurse, or a piece of technology. In fact, Anne and other patients often displayed an impressive level of expertise and rhetoric from a biomedical perspective regarding their diabetes, for example, when analyzing graphs of blood sugar levels. It seemed that Anne and other patients at the clinic in Aarhus had formed a certain understanding of their diabetes and how it should be treated.

This is, of course, not the same as arguing that Anne would consistently treat her diabetes accordingly (as evident, for instance, from her overeating of candy), but she still displayed certainty as to what she considered to be accurate and factual of her condition and its treatment. Her understandings were greatly aligned with those of the healthcare personnel she consulted with at the clinic in Aarhus; a stark contrast to the clinic, for example, in Giza. This was so, I argue, as Anne and others frequenting the clinic in Aarhus had been trained through years of consultations, blood sugar measurements, the utilization of insulin devices, apps, and so-called "camps" and "schools" for children, to think of their diabetes in certain ways. Anne's nurse did not have to visibly "govern" (Miller and Rose 2008) Anne in any way in relation to her condition; she had already been "governed" and was in tune with the objectives of the healthcare personnel to take care of her diabetes in specific ways. "I know my diabetes better than anyone else," she stated while confidently measuring her own blood sugar levels, adjusting her insulin pump, and downloading relevant apps for her phone.

Even though the above example of Anne may seem taken out of context, I draw on it here in order to provide the reader with just that; a view into the context from which Novo drew their understandings of proper diabetes care specifically and proper medical conduct generally. By drawing on the above example of Anne, I wish to finally problematize the ways in which Novo attempted to transfer such understandings into an Egyptian social, political, and medical context. Albeit the supposedly good intentions of Novo to better diabetes treatment in Egypt, the effects of enforcing such specific understandings on those diagnosed with type-2 diabetes had the contrary overall effect of adding to the uncertainties that constituted their treatment paths. The enforcement by Novo Nordisk of what they perceived, for example, as a universal set of medical ethics onto an Egyptian context, I argue, rather undermined individuals and their personal experiences and struggles of living with type-2 diabetes in Egypt.

In summary, what Anne knew of her diabetes seemed attuned with that of her healthcare providers. In the words of her nurse, Anne was displaying a "high level of compliance." In contrast, the certainty with which healthcare personnel in Cairo promoted specific etiologies and treatments did not bring about the ability to "govern" the behavior of Cairene patients; rather, such attempts at bringing about a certainty of diabetes and its treatment paths was met with a great many uncertainties.

I wish to end this chapter with a couple of notes on trust. Sociologist Jack Barbalet has argued on the nature of trust, "Trust [...] is a means of overcoming the absence of evidence, without benefit of the standard of rational proof, which is required to sustain relationships between persons or between a person and a social artifact" (Barbalet 2009:367). Whereas patients such as Anne at the clinic in Aarhus clearly displayed general trust in information, people, and social artifacts (such as her insulin pump), this was not generally the case among the people that I was working with in Cairo. Accepting the notion of a prescription in a legal sense, for example, meant also accepting and trusting in the expertise of doctors and thus "overcoming the absence of evidence."

Barbarlet further argues, "The value of trust is especially apparent to those who face improbity and deception" (Barbalet 2009:367).

As I hope I have made evident by now, to people in Cairo, trusting a great many others was often perceived as risky business, precisely because the possibility of facing "improbity and deception" was very real. This has been made evident throughout the book, for example, in the frequent stories and personal experiences of medical misconduct (Chapter 2) as well as in the stories and personal experiences of contaminations or sudden shortages of foods and pharmaceutical drugs (Chapters 3 and 4). Barbalet elaborates on the nature of trust that it is "based on expectation, not deliberative calculation" (Barbalet 2009:378). In other words, trust points to future situations, "outcomes that have not occurred at the time of the choice to act or trust" (Barbalet 2009:378).

The uncertainties intrinsic to many spheres of everyday life in Cairo, I hold, made people cautious to expect certain outcomes of others. As opposed to succumbing to what was perceived as an illusion of certainty promoted, for example, by doctors and authorities, people aimed to maintain a state of uncertainty as this was perceived a safer way to move forward in many spheres of everyday life.

Philosopher Georg Simmel has argued that without a general display of trust in others societies would "disintegrate" (Simmel 2004:178–9). Trust, in the arguments of Simmel, in other words appears to be essential for social cohesion. I wish to finally argue here, in contrast, that maintaining a state of uncertainty appeared to be essential for social cohesion among people in Cairo throughout my years of research. The people I worked with thus emphasized the importance of facing and resisting structural uncertainties by upholding a sense of uncertainty themselves; persistently raising questions, for example, about the narratives of politics or etiologies of diabetes. However, even though people insisted on maintaining such a state of uncertainty, for example to protect themselves from medical misconduct, the uncertainty was also fundamentally linked to experiences of *ḍaghṭ* and subsequently to the onset or worsening of type-2 diabetes.

Before turning to summarize this final chapter, I wish to emphasize here that trust, of course, was prevailing within many social relations in many different spheres of everyday life in Cairo. However, throughout this book I have chosen to focus on those spheres in which uncertainty and mistrust rather characterized the relations as this seemed also to overall characterize and form understandings of type-2 diabetes and its treatment.

The Novo Care Center, Continued ... (September 2015)

A man in his 50s enters the center. He walks quickly toward Nadia, with his wife a few steps behind him. The man is very upset, and he speaks to Nadia in an angry tone. He wants a NovoPen, and he wants it now! Apparently, he takes two types of insulin; he has a pen for one type, but not for the other.

"I have to use a syringe for the other," he says, "and I am fed up with the syringe!"

Nadia explains in a calm tone that there are no more pens.

"We ran out of pens," she says, "*Mafīsh*, I do not have any pens here." Nadia points to the storage room next to us, door open, room clearly empty. "The pens are at the airport," she finally explains.

The man starts shouting at Nadia. He is tired and sick from running around, all over the city, trying to track down a pen.

"Please be patient," Nadia says.

The man angrily shouts back at her, "Is it you or me who has to take the insulin?" Nadia sighs, and repeats once again that there is nothing she can do. She leans back in her chair, hands in her lap. She does not break eye contact with the man. He then starts shouting at Novo Nordisk.

"This is a bad company," he says.

Nadia interrupts him, "There is nothing wrong with the company. It's not the company's fault that the pens are still at the airport." The man finally demands to speak to Nadia's superior. "That's fine, that's no problem," Nadia says. She gets up, and enters the back office, calling Ayman, her superior, on the phone.

I can hear her discuss the situation with Ayman, before returning to the desk with the phone. She hands the phone to the man. The man greets Ayman. It is mostly Ayman talking on the other end. The man throws in a few comments, such as, "I am a tired man," and "I can barely walk."

"*Il-balad waskha*, the country is dirty," he finally comments on Ayman's monologue. He hangs up the phone, and hands it to Nadia. He looks at her for a couple of seconds, and then bursts out laughing. Nadia and the man's wife start laughing as well. The man finally throws his hands up into the air, as if accepting that there is nothing he or anyone else can do to change the situation. Laughingly, he and his wife leave the center.

I ask Nadia about the pens. She tells me that Novo cannot get the pens released from the customs office at the airport.

"Something with money and politics," she mumbles, clearly not willing to elaborate much. She explains that they ran out of pens three days ago. "And not just this office – all of Cairo ..." I ask her if it happens often.

"It's rare, but it happens," she says. She tells me that the man does not like to use regular syringes because they break easily, and they hurt. She adds, "A lot of diabetics are nervous and easily get upset, but we still have to deal with them in a good way." I nod, impressed that Nadia was so calm through the whole ordeal. She shows me a list of names on her desk. "I currently have 15 people I have to call when the pen is back, last time I had to call more than 100 people."

A woman enters the office. She walks straight up to Nadia's desk.

"Is the pen here or still ...?" she asks.

"Still ..." Nadia says.

The woman sighs, mumbling quietly, "*Mushkila*, it's a problem."

She leaves the center again. Throughout the day, several other people enter the office to get hold of a pen. Nadia adds them to the growing list of people to call, telling them to try in "a few days," "toward the end of the month," or "perhaps next week."

Summary

Several high-ranking employees within Novo Nordisk in Egypt mentioned the challenges of passing goods through the Egyptian customs office at the airport in Cairo in ways considered legal by Novo Nordisk. Put differently, Novo refused to bribe customs officers, and this occasionally meant that pens, insulin, and other goods were not released on the Egyptian market in time to prevent shortages such as the one depicted above. As outlined also in the previous chapters, reports of corrupt officials are frequent in Egypt. When I was first writing up this chapter, headlines were, in fact, circulating in several Egyptian newspapers specifically addressing the corruption at the customs office at the international airport in Cairo.

The above encounter at the Novo Care Center illustrates yet another attempt by Novo Nordisk to enforce certain ideas or policies in Cairo, though in this case the policy was related to proper corporate conduct, rather than to proper medical conduct as such. Throughout this chapter, I have presented various attempts by Novo Nordisk to implement certain policies with the purpose of improving business opportunities, as well as improving diabetes care in Egypt (from the perspective of Novo Nordisk anyway). As evident throughout the analysis above, these policies all carried specific objectives and "technologies," such as reducing the "over-prescribing" and "self-prescribing" of medicine by enforcing legal prescriptions, or remaining financially transparent by insisting on not bribing officials. Yet, these policies had effects that I suspect were not intended by Novo Nordisk, such as the delay of insulin treatment for recently diagnosed customers (due to the enforcements of prescriptions), or the general shortage of products (due to their refusal to pay bribes).

"We have to alter what they think," Aaliyah stated at the beginning of this chapter, referring to Novo Nordisk as "We," and Egyptians (both those with diabetes, and, as it turned out, officials more generally as well) as "they." Yet, this was easier said than done, as neither patients, doctors, nor health officials were simply compliant or adherent to Novo's policies or ways of doing business. Rather, they faced these attempts with a display of resistance and a broad range of questions. I argue that this resistance essentially came out of a lack of trust in authorities and expertise. As unfolded also in the previous chapters, past experiences, for example, of medical misconduct had taught people to stay cautious in relation to authorities and their advice.

Throughout the chapters, I have raised the empirical question of why the etiology of "diabesity" was not so readily accepted among people with type-2 diabetes in Cairo, despite the consistent promotion of this particular etiology by pharmaceutical companies such as Novo Nordisk, as well as by Egyptian healthcare personnel in general. Based on the analysis presented above, I argue that reasons for this resistance can be found in the uncertainty experienced and generated by people in Cairo over attributes such as certainty or trust in authorities (and their potential expertise). In order for facts to become facts in Cairo (for example, in relation to type-2 diabetes), people needed to trust in information, certain people, and technologies in ways which commonly they did not. For this reason, the etiology of "diabesity" was not so readily accepted, despite great attempts by doctors, Novo Nordisk, and others to transform the understanding of type-2 diabetes and diabetes care.

I choose to end this chapter with the above empirical encounter to emphasize the ways in which people in Cairo generally displayed a very firm understanding of type-2 diabetes as related to *ḍaghṭ*, and not to obesity, yet, as is also evident throughout the past chapters, this did not mean that they did not follow any of the advice given to them by their doctors. Therefore, people such as the man in the above still showed great frustration when they could not access certain medicine, raising questions as to, for example, the trustworthiness of Novo Nordisk ("*il-company*") and the country at large ("*il-ballad*"). Whereas Novo refused to pay bribes as a way, I suspect, to appear trustworthy to customers and investors, this very act had in fact the opposite effect on the man described above. He and others were, once again, confirmed in their reluctance to trust in authorities and companies such as Novo Nordisk and their ability, for example, to provide a steady supply of medicine and medical technologies. As evident in the above example, this left the man in question suggesting that the company had hidden agendas, was covering up information, and, for reasons unknown, not releasing the NovoPen to him specifically. In an attempt to promote certainty in their products and in the company at large, Novo left the people of Cairo, once again, with great uncertainty as to the supply of drugs, but also as to the general agendas of a multinational pharmaceutical industry.

Notes

1 2 EGP was approximately equivalent to 0.1 USD as of October 2018.
2 Parts of this ethnographic vignette have previously been published in the book chapter, "Risky notes" (see Thorsen 2020).

References

Appadurai, Arjun. 1988. *The Social Life of Things: Commodities in Cultural Perspective*. Cambridge University Press.

Barbalet, Jack. 2009. A Characterization of Trust, and Its Consequences. *Theory and Society* 38(4): 367–382.

Cramer, J. A., Á. Benedict, N. Muszbek, A. Keskinaslan, and Z. M. Khan. 2008. The Significance of Compliance and Persistence in the Treatment of Diabetes, Hypertension and Dyslipidaemia: A Review. *International Journal of Clinical Practice* 62(1): 76–87.

Dewey, John. 1929. *The Quest for Certainty*. Capricorn Books.

Foucault, Michel. 1991. *The Foucault Effect: Studies in Governmentality with Two Lectures by and an Interview with Michel Foucault*. Graham Burchell, Colin Gordon, and Peter Miller, eds. University of Chicago Press.

Geest, Sjaak van der, Anita Hardon, and Susan R. Whyte. 1996. The Anthropology of Pharmaceuticals: A Biographical Approach. *Annual Review of Anthropology* 25(1): 153–178.

Miller, Peter, and Nikolas Rose. 2008. *Governing the Present: Administering Economic, Social and Personal Life*. Peter Miller, and Nikolas Rose, eds. Polity.

Mitchell, Timothy. 2002. *Rule of Experts: Egypt, Techno-Politics, Modernity*. University of California Press.

Moran-Thomas, Amy. 2019. What Is Communicable? Unaccounted Injuries and "Catching" Diabetes in an Illegible Epidemic. *Cultural Anthropology* 34(4): 471–502.
Simmel, Georg. 2004. *The Philosophy of Money*. Routledge.
Thorsen, Mille K. 2020. Risky Notes: Reading Tense Situations in Cairo in 2015. *In Anthropology Inside Out: Fieldworkers Taking Note*. A. Andersen, L. Dalsgård, M. L. Kusk, et al., eds. Pp. 135–150. Sean Kingston Publishing.
Whyte, Susan R. 1997. *Questioning Misfortune: The Pragmatics of Uncertainty in Eastern Uganda*. Cambridge University Press.

7 Final Notes

During my first months of fieldwork in Cairo in 2015, I persistently questioned the people that I worked with about the processes ahead of us before visiting, for example, doctors, hospitals, or any other kind of bureaucratic institution: How is one commonly diagnosed with type-2 diabetes? Where does one go when experiencing certain symptoms? What does the doctor commonly do when examining the patient? Which papers do you need in order to retrieve the free insulin? Who has to sign the paper? What will happen next? In other words, I tried to lay out the plot of the story before setting out to collect it.

"*Hanshūf*, we'll see," was the most common response to my questions, accompanied by laughter at my bewilderment and my attempt to map out the process ahead of our endeavors. Evident throughout the chapters of this book, making sense of type-2 diabetes in a Cairene context turned out not to be related so much to the construction of coherent narratives of illness as it was to fragmented stories of experiences of *ḍaghṭ* and the uncertainties intrinsic to those experiences: stories of red chicken, white chicken, sugar shortages, Sovaldi medicine and its cancerous effects, love, marriage, grief, corruption, and a range of other stories filled the pages of my notebooks – all constituting a mosaic of responses given to me when raising questions on the topic of type-2 diabetes.

With this book I suggest that digging into such stories is one place to begin to improve type-2 diabetes care in Egypt – by acknowledging the experiences of those diagnosed with the condition, not merely in order to tap into the understanding of the local, but as a way to recognize that the high prevalence of type-2 diabetes in Egypt, and in this region at large, relate to much more complex issues than merely an excess consumption of food and calories.

Throughout this book, I have argued that sentiments of uncertainty carry a long history in Egypt as a political tool used to control

DOI: 10.4324/9781003327684-7

the population; however, I have also illustrated how uncertainty was invoked by the general population in Cairo during my years of research to resist and protect themselves from political, social, and medical harm. However, paradoxically, such uncertainties of, for example, political narratives and medical treatment were also perceived among those diagnosed with the condition and their loved ones to cause experiences of *ḍaghṭ* and subsequently type-2 diabetes. Treatment thus came to revolve primarily around relieving those suffering from type-2 diabetes from experiences of *ḍaghṭ*, as opposed to adding additional *ḍaghṭ*, for example, through dieting, exercising, or other means.

These understandings of type-2 diabetes, albeit biomedically acknowledged as related to the onset of type-2 diabetes, were persistently undermined by Egyptian healthcare personnel promoting exclusively an etiology of "diabesity" in relation to the condition. This etiology was supported also by Novo Nordisk who was greatly involved with diabetes care within the country. Overall, this book has aimed to illustrate the ways in which biomedical research may point to multiple etiologies of type-2 diabetes; however, the complexities of these different etiologies disappear and transform into a simpler story of "diabesity," both in international medical guidelines and policies, but also among healthcare personnel in Cairo. Nonetheless, I wish to raise the question here – if people in Cairo were easily "governed" (Miller and Rose 2008) to conform to type-2 diabetes treatment in ways promoted, for example, by Novo Nordisk or local healthcare personnel, would it resolve the "problem" (Spector and Kitsuse 2001) of type-2 diabetes in Egypt?

Based on the arguments presented throughout this book, I feel confident when arguing that it would not as long as structural conditions and inequities on a global and local scale are not addressed: in what ways do the policies of the International Monetary Fund or the desire of multinational pharmaceutical companies to gather certain data within the public healthcare sector, for example, contribute to the prevalence and poor treatment of type-2 diabetes in Egypt? For diabetes treatment and prevention strategies to better succeed, I hold, such questions must be considered and included as part of the overall story of type-2 diabetes.

Turning to the closing pages of this book, I wish to end this story of type-2 diabetes in Egypt by acknowledging the simultaneous strains and beauties of this country and its uncertainties, with hopes that we can all insist on raising questions and doubting that which we think we know of type-2 diabetes.

References

Miller, Peter, and Nikolas Rose. 2008. *Governing the Present: Administering Economic, Social and Personal Life*. Peter Miller, and Nikolas Rose, eds. Polity.

Spector, Malcolm, and John I. Kitsuse. 2001. *Constructing Social Problems*. Transaction Publishers.

Epilogue

"In the movie the main character takes everyone in this building as hostages. Have you seen it?" Mohamed looks at me as we are trying to navigate our way down the busy corridors. We are in the Mugamma, a massive governmental building just off Tahrir Square in downtown Cairo. It's June 2015 and I need an extension of my visa. The building is bustling with activity. I tell Mohamed that I haven't seen the movie.

"It sounds horrible," I add while tailing him closely down the hallway.

"No, it's a comedy," Mohamed says, turning his face slightly my way. "*Il-'irhāb wa il-kabāb*, terrorism and kebab. It's the name of the movie." For a few seconds I ponder over the title of the movie and how one makes a comedy about terror, but then my attention is directed toward navigating the busy hallways. Men, women, children, young and old. The corridors are full of people moving in different directions, entering different rooms, stopping to ask someone for something, sitting on chairs, in corners, or on the floor. Resting. Waiting.

Some are filling out paperwork, others are sleeping or feeding their babies under layers of clothes. It's early morning, but already extremely hot. The air is oppressive, thick with dust and the smell of sweat; it sticks in my nostrils and on my skin. We take a sharp turn. Mohamed is keeping a steady pace. The darkened corridors all look similar – windows on each side, with workers behind them, people queuing up. The floors and walls are peppered with dirty, weathered, broken tiles. I am grateful to have Mohamed by my side, someone who knows his way around. Not literally. He keeps asking for directions. But he knows his way around. Around Cairo, around the system. I stay close to him as he leads me to the right, then to the left, and then somewhere, I already forgot where. We are pushing our way through the crowds. I hear many dialects of Arabic and many languages I don't recognize.

It is getting more and more crowded as we move our way farther into the building. I notice a small note in English above a window, "Refugees." A huge group of people are gathered in front of it, pushing each other around, shouting in shrill voices. Babies are crying. We pass by the group, down a different corridor. Moving forward.

An old man appears from within the crowd. He comes up to me, waiving a visa application form under my nose.

"Five pounds," he shouts as if he is selling mangos outside in the street. Mohamed looks at him and then glances quickly back at me.

"You can get the form for free if we just find the right person ..." Mohamed says. He is speaking in a loud voice, trying to make himself heard above everyone else. I ignore the old man.

We reach Window 38. It says "Tourist" in English on a small note above it. Mohamed pushes his way to the front, asking where I can apply for an extension of my visa. The woman behind the counter tells us to go to Window 12. We push our way down the corridor to Window 12. Once again, Mohamed pushes his way to the front. The woman behind the counter tells him that I need to get an application form from Window 38. We go back to Window 38. Another old man stops me on our way. He is selling pens. I decide to buy one to support his business. He gives me a red pen. "Two pounds."

Mohamed gets me an application form from Window 38. I fill out the form with the red pen, writing up against a wall. People are pushing me around, all trying to find the right windows and forms for whatever business brings them here. I complete filling out the application and go back to Window 12. The woman behind the counter looks at me.

"You have to use a black pen," she says as she refuses to accept the application. I grab the form and look at Mohamed. We go back to Window 38 to get a new form. On our way back, I pass the old man selling pens. I tell him that the woman didn't accept my application because of the red pen.

He looks at me and says, "Yeah, they don't accept red pens. You need a black pen." He holds out a handful of black pens, red pens sticking out of his pocket. "Two pounds," he says. Slightly annoyed, I ask him why he would sell me the red pen in the first place. I decide to give up on the conversation, and instead ask him for a black pen. "Two pounds."

Mohamed quickly returns with a new application. I fill out the form standing on the same spot as before, writing up against the wall. The black pen doesn't work. I try scribbling with it on another piece of paper, to no avail. Annoyed, I fetch out a pen from my bag and start filling out the form. I quickly finish and return to Window number 12.

The woman behind the counter tells us to go to Window 5 to buy stamps to pay for the extension of the visa – 3.10 pounds worth of stamps. Mohamed and I empty our pockets to find the exact amount in change. We manage and go to Window 5. We buy my stamps after much waiting and pushing around. I ask Mohamed if we should put the stamps on the application, so we won't lose them. He shakes his head.

"Maybe they will say we didn't do it the right way … Better have them do it. Bureaucracy, you know?" he says. He smiles at me. We return to Window 12. We push our way to the front and hand the woman behind the counter my application. Everyone is trying to push their way to the front. The woman puts the stamps on the application and then writes today's date at the bottom.

"You have to hand it in at Window 38," she says as she hands the application back to me. She is speaking in a loud and clear voice behind the glass window. I turn my ear toward her to better hear her. I nod at her instructions and turn to Mohamed. We glance at each other and then move our way back down the corridor to Window 38.

I try to push my way to the front to get the attention of the woman working behind the counter. She is drinking tea and talking to a colleague, both laughing. After some time, the woman turns to face me behind the window. I try to hand her my application. She gives me a blank stare.

"I am closed for the rest of the day," she says, refusing to accept my application. I glance over at a sign hanging next to the window: "8am–1pm." It's only 9:30am. I point to the sign. The woman looks at me as if she couldn't care less.

"I already took in too many applications today. Come back tomorrow," she says. She immediately turns around and starts chatting with her colleague again.

Mohamed and I move our way out of the building. Once outside, we find a spot in the shade.

"She probably wanted some *baqshīsh*, a tip," Mohamed says. I look at him and only now realize that I should have paid the woman a small bribe. Or to put it in Mohamed's terms, "a tip."

"You know, I went to get a driver's license last week and I wanted to do it 'the right way,'" Mohamed makes quotation marks in the air, "So, I went to the right office and everything. And I was the only one there who wasn't granted a license. Probably because I decided not to pay anyone in advance." We sit for a while. Mohamed then says, "I think I will just buy it from this guy I know in the street."

I return the following day to hand in my visa application. Mohamed has work, so I am on my own. I show up before the building is open for business and queue up with all the workers. A band has set up a small stage next to the queue and is rocking away, playing their music. Huge amplifiers are blasting the sound all over the square. It's only 8am. A live rock concert for all the administrative workers. A man taps me on my shoulder.

"Women don't have to wait in line," he says and points to the entrance way down the queue. I see women entering before all the men. I tell him thanks and hurry down to the entrance. I quickly enter the building and find my way through detectors and corridors. I get lost twice – first, going to a wrong floor, then making a wrong turn down one of the corridors. But I finally find Window 38. The woman from yesterday is waiting behind the counter. I hand her my application and passport. She accepts it.

"Come back in three days at 1pm exactly," she instructs me. "Your visa will be ready then."

"Here?" I ask.

"No. Window 12," she says.

Three days later, I return for my third visit. I now know my way to Windows 12 and 38 just fine. I pass quickly through the building. Fewer people are here today than during my last two visits but I feel confident that the woman told me to come back today. I find the corridor of Windows 12 and 38. No one is here. I walk around, searching the hallways. Finally, I find a young man sleeping in one of the offices, resting his head on the desk. I can see him through Window 74. I knock on the window, and he looks up. I explain that I am supposed to pick up my passport today. Now, actually, at 1pm, "exactly, *bāṣabṭ*," I add. He looks at me. His eyes still seem asleep.

"No, we are closed today," he says. I look at him confused.

"When did you leave your passport here?" he then asks. I tell him I left it here three days ago. "No, you are supposed to come back the following day to pick up your passport," he explains, sighing deeply. I look at him in vain.

"But I need my passport ..." I say. I start getting a bit nervous thinking about my passport, already considering how to get a new one from the embassy.

The young man sighs once again, visibly annoyed.

"Okay okay," he says. "Come ..."

He walks behind the windows all the way down the corridor and opens a door to the office. He tells me to enter. He grabs two black garbage bags from underneath a counter and empties the contents of both of them on one of the desks. Passports of many nationalities fall out in huge piles.

"It should be here somewhere," he points, gesturing that I can try to find it myself. He leaves me to it.

I start rummaging through the passports. After a while, I start sorting the passports into piles according to nationality. After about ten minutes, I find my own passport. I check for the visa, considering the option that the woman didn't process my visa at all, but I got the extension. I smile, almost raising my hands above my head to cheer in victory. I look around. The young man is nowhere to be found. I leave the big pile of passports behind, half of them organized neatly on the desk, the other half still in a huge messy pile. I hurry through the corridors and out of the building, left with a profound sense that I am finally getting the hang of it. Better at finding my own way around.

Index

For Product Safety Concerns and Information please contact our EU
representative GPSR@taylorandfrancis.com
Taylor & Francis Verlag GmbH, Kaufingerstraße 24, 80331 München, Germany

www.ingramcontent.com/pod-product-compliance
Ingram Content Group UK Ltd.
Pitfield, Milton Keynes, MK11 3LW, UK
UKHW021307260926
475702UK00048B/806
9781032328669